W9-CKL-302

WITHDRAWN

Stupid Reasons People Die

An Ingenious Plot
for Defusing Deadly Diseases

by

John Corso, M.D.

Copyright © 2007 by High Lakes Press, LLC
All rights reserved. No part of the material protected by this copyright notice may be reproduced or utilized in any form or by any means, electronic or mechanical, including photocopying, recording or by any informational storage and retrieval system without written permission from the copyright owner.

www.highlakespress.com

*Publisher's Cataloging-in-Publication
(Provided by Quality Books, Inc.)*

Corso, John, 1955-
    Stupid reasons people die : an ingenious plot for defusing deadly diseases / by John Corso.
    p. cm.
    Includes bibliographical references and index.
    LCCN 2006937973
    ISBN-13: 978-0-9789922-1-7
    ISBN-10: 0-9789922-1-0
    ISBN-13: 978-0-9789922-0-0
    ISBN-10: 0-9789922-0-2

    1. Self-care, Health. 2. Medicine, Preventive—
Popular works.   I. Title.

RA776.95.C67 2007   613
                               QBI06-600717

Cover Art Design and Book Illustrations: Mark Blackwell
blackwellart@gmail.com

Manuscript Editor: Vicki Grant
writebend@aol.com

Copy Editing: Cynthia Stark
copyeditpro@bendbroadband.com
www.copyeditpro.com

Contents

Important for You to Know

The information provided in this book contains the opinions and ideas of the author, and the content is general and educational in nature. The author is not engaged in rendering medical, therapeutic, or other advice, instruction, or services in this publication. If you purchased or otherwise came into possession of this book for the purpose of obtaining personal advice of any kind or nature whatsoever, you should return this book and obtain a refund of any consideration you paid to obtain it and disregard any portion of the book you have read.

Information and opinions offered here are based on a small subset of the medical knowledge available at the time of publication. No medical action or decision should be made solely on this information. Instead, readers should consult health professionals on all matters related to their health and well-being, and readers who fail to consult appropriate health professionals assume all the risk of any injuries.

The author does not warrant the contents or accuracy of this publication or the sources quoted or otherwise referenced including other books, articles, Internet sites, or any other media, and specifically disclaims, to the fullest extent permitted by law, any and all warranties, express or implied, of any kind or nature whatsoever. The author is not responsible for errors or omissions. Furthermore, the author will not be liable to you for any damages, claims, demands, or causes of action, direct or indirect, special, incidental, consequential, or punitive, related to your diagnosis, treatment, or your healthcare decisions.

~~~

Introduction

Our healthcare system exists in a state of crisis.

It took a radical change in my own medical practice before I fully appreciated the tragic consequences of relying on this system to keep us alive and well.

Without malice or intent, it plays Russian Roulette with patient lives, because it is primarily designed around solving problems, not preventing them. Physicians must compress their services into a ten-minute diagnosis and treatment regimen.

Patients feel compelled to jump through hoops for "permission" to get those ten minutes. The general public is unaware of advancements that finally make it possible to capture and arrest the diseases most responsible for cutting life short.

Of course, we serve patients best by helping them avoid catastrophic illness. Yet our current system is a barrier to just that. The devil lurks in the details of myriad signs, symptoms, behaviors, and nuances that are rarely uncovered in the imposed ten-minute window.

Patients arrive with serious problems that often could have been averted with education and early intervention. And this defeats the point of healthcare. Here we are with remarkable knowledge, tools, and opportunities to get *ahead* of problems. Instead, we chase after them.

For a long time, I ignored any medical journal with *prevention* in the title. Fine publications, but the word "prevention" put me to sleep. For most of us, prevention doesn't refer to action, but to a *do-nothing* or *stop-doing* position.

"Don't eat the whole cheesecake!"

"Don't sit on your butt all day!"

"Don't play with matches."

Good advice, but only the tip of the prevention iceberg. True prevention is about *doing*. It's a hunt, a vigilant, proactive search and seizure. It means an extensive investigation to find diseases lurking in patients, even in those currently enjoying glowing health. It's making sure they *stay* that way.

I began weighing the pros and cons of a medical practice that would not rely on the system to dictate the level of care or amount of time I could give to patients. I wanted a practice that gave prevention a new meaning.

Taking direct, focused action *now* by using the state-of-the-art in health screening technology, and using the best available treatments when needed, is the key to stopping potential killers and sustaining or restoring health.

It was a leap of faith within a healthcare system that is neither willing nor able to invest in high-level preventive care. The unknowable factor was how patients would respond to care that went beyond what was included in their benefits package—that required a change in perspective—that meant being an assertive collaborator instead of a submissive patient. It was astonishing and affirming how quickly patients stepped up to the plate.

My practice today is the result of a long-held conviction that each of us is responsible for our own healthcare. When we abdicate that responsibility to insurers, employers, policy makers, and bureaucrats, we put our lives in the hands of institutions that do not exist to serve us. I consider that a very stupid reason to die.

I would like to help you avoid that fate by arming you with insight, information, and inspiration that puts *you* in control of the content, quality, and cost of your healthcare. It is not difficult or time-consuming; you just need to be ready to look at things in a different light.

First, I'll ask you to face the truth of how your own biases, our healthcare system, and society all conspire to keep you in a passive role.

This sets the stage for Part Two, where a survival guide arms you with state-of-the-art methods for outsmarting the diseases most likely to cross the paths of you and your loved ones. New medical breakthroughs will continually change the opportunities for early disease detection and intervention, but you will be right there on the front lines, primed for action.

～～～

PART ONE

WHAT ARE YOU THINKING?

*"There are only a few stupid reasons people die—
they just happen to kill a whole lot of people."*

Chapter 1

Rumors, Tumors and Baby Boomers

Ed was having a *very* good night. It may have been a freezing Michigan evening in the dead of winter, but Ed was glowing. He had just bowled a perfect 300 for the benefit of his team, the third perfect game of his life.

He had been bowling for decades, but *these* three scores were all hallmarks of the past two years, as was his induction into the Kalamazoo Bowling Hall of Fame. Life was great. Ed was at his peak.

Ten more pins went their separate ways as he nailed another strike on the fourth frame of the next game. Returning to his chair, he suddenly knew something was terribly wrong. Then, nothing.

Friends and family watched their Kalamazoo hero clutch his chest and collapse. A tiny blood clot had suddenly formed in Ed's heart. His life simply stopped.

John Ritter's darling daughter was celebrating her 5th birthday, just a few days prior to her dad's 55th. Her famous father was busy, preparing to tape the latest episode of his hit television series, *8 Simple Rules for Dating My Teenage Daughter*.

While working on the set, he began to feel ill. Things quickly went from bad to worse and Mr. Ritter was rushed to St. Joseph's, the same Burbank hospital where he was born. Several hours later, as a team of surgeons struggled to repair his torn aorta, he died on the operating table.

The sudden tear that ended John Ritter's life was reportedly due to a heart defect, an undetected problem Mr. Ritter may have had since birth.

Ed's story made the national news because in the midst of personal glory he dropped dead. John received even greater coverage because he was well known to most Americans.

Every day, the lives of average, healthy-looking folks come to an abrupt end, sending shock waves of misery through the lives of their loved ones. Their stories may lack the tragic irony or celebrity status to make them newsworthy, but for every John Ritter, there are a thousand John Does.

As I write this, the first baby boomers are just hitting 60, and the average life span in America is up to 78 years. And that's great, since life expectancy was only 40 years just a century ago.

Yet it's a harsh statistical fact that in every group, *somebody* has to fall below the average. This means that for all the spry characters who make it to their 80s and 90s, an equivalent number of unlucky souls die long before Medicare ever kicks in.

We've all seen it. A father dies suddenly of a massive heart attack. A mother wastes away from cancer. End of story. No more holidays, soccer games, or school plays to share with the family. Someone else must walk their daughters down the aisle. Show up to your next high school reunion, and you're sure to hear about a few more.

Here's the tragedy: Many of these people die in the prime of life from common medical conditions *we already know* how to find and fix.

How could this happen? In most cases, it happens because no one looked for or treated the problem the right way, in the right place, at the right time.

Devastated friends and relatives, watching a loved one die, can't help asking if something could have prevented this life from ending so soon. Whether the patient is suffocating from congestive heart failure or battling a cancer consuming their body, the answer is often a heart-breaking "yes." It's terrible to realize that someone you loved might still have been with you.

Every year, tens of thousands of people "slip through the cracks" and pay the ultimate price. And it's not that we don't care! Both the health-conscious and the "worried well" in America spend billions of dollars on products that promise to keep them healthy or ensure a long life.

No-Fat! • *All-Natural!* • *Lite-Lite-Lite!*

If a fraction of this energy and money was applied to truly effective screening, prevention, and treatment, death could be postponed for tens of thousands of men and women.

There are countless "stay healthy" books to guide you through myriad dietary and lifestyle changes, herbal and vitamin cures, and other instant miracles to ensure your health and longevity. This is not one of them.

Even the books with good advice on healthy living don't seem to inspire and sustain meaningful changes. They just leave most readers feeling guilty. Often, it seems impossible for busy people with too many demands and not enough time to redesign their lifestyle.

Not that cutting back on junk food or taking time to exercise are bad ideas; they're not. But here's the irony. Even if you pull it off—exercise every day, eat only salad, fish and tofu, take vitamins, meditate, and grow your own organic vegetables, you will only increase your chances of avoiding a preventable early death by a tiny percentage.

In fact, if every citizen in this country ran five miles a day and never again ate cholesterol-laden food, there would still be millions of people like Ed, dying for stupid reasons, dying because of heart attacks, strokes, cancers, and other diseases that could have been detected and stopped.

This book is about *real* results. And real results for living longer don't come from good intentions and superhuman discipline. They come from being smart about identifying and treating the things most likely to kill *you*.

It's not difficult to avoid the most common killers if you accept that reducing your chances of dying young is worth a little effort and money. That is what this book will help you do. Minimal scare tactics, no false promises, and no reasons to feel guilty.

When people die prematurely, it's rarely because they're lazy, simple-minded, or have a death wish. It's because they're misled. But while it may not be their fault, they *are* part of the problem. If you are an average, forty-plus American, you're most likely focusing your efforts to be healthy on the wrong things. Most of us plow headlong into harm's way because of some basic things we fail to do and because of one thing we should never have allowed in the first place. I will bet that:

▶ **You are not getting all the right tests to see if you have a life-threatening medical time bomb waiting to go off.**

▶ **You are not taking the medicine, supplements, or other treatments that can defuse that bomb.**

▶ **You are not separating useful health information from the hype, partial facts, and plain nonsense you get from the news media.**

▶ **But you *are* allowing accountants, bureaucrats, policy makers, and politicians to make major healthcare decisions for you, perhaps unknowingly.**

Medical issues fascinate many of us and affect the health of all of us. They also make juicy headlines, whether it's Mad Cow prime rib, the dangers of Phen-Fen, or the latest Avian Flu scare. Yet *this* simple fact never makes the daily news:

Your number one, greatest risk of dying is from a disease that can be prevented or successfully treated.

Apparently, this crucial message isn't considered newsworthy. Of course, there are a million ways to die. A meteorite could fall from the sky and end my life in an instant. An inoperable brain tumor could kill me in a few months, or I might just get onto the wrong plane at the wrong time. I hope to avoid all three, but I don't worry about them. These possibilities and thousands like them are unavoidable, incurable, or random tragedies.

Most of the time, however, death is a dreary, predictable intruder. It comes in the guise of some health condition that can be detected and arrested before it claims its victim. Yet, it slips in easily and frequently, picking off friends and family *because we aren't paying attention!*

If there were hundreds of complicated things we need to do to avoid such disaster, there might be an excuse for not taking action. But, here's the frustration: There are only a few stupid reasons people die; they just happen to kill a whole lot of people.

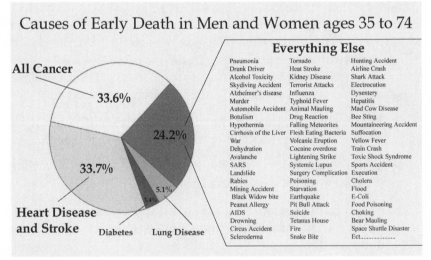

Causes of Early Death in Men and Women ages 35 to 74

All Cancer

33.6%

24.2%

33.7%

5.1%

Heart Disease and Stroke   Diabetes   Lung Disease

Everything Else

Pneumonia	Tornado	Hunting Accident
Drunk Driver	Heat Stroke	Airline Crash
Alcohol Toxicity	Kidney Disease	Shark Attack
Skydiving Accident	Terrorist Attacks	Electrocution
Alzheimer's disease	Influenza	Dysentery
Murder	Typhoid Fever	Hepatitis
Automobile Accident	Animal Mauling	Mad Cow Disease
Botulism	Drug Reaction	Bee Sting
Hypothermia	Falling Meteorites	Mountaineering Accident
Cirrhosis of the Liver	Flesh Eating Bacteria	Suffocation
War	Volcanic Eruption	Yellow Fever
Dehydration	Cocaine overdose	Train Crash
Avalanche	Lightening Strike	Toxic Shock Syndrome
SARS	Systemic Lupus	Sports Accident
Landslide	Surgery Complication	Execution
Rabies	Poisoning	Cholera
Mining Accident	Starvation	Flood
Black Widow bite	Earthquake	E-Coli
Peanut Allergy	Pit Bull Attack	Food Poisoning
AIDS	Suicide	Choking
Drowning	Tetanus House	Bear Mauling
Circus Accident	Fire	Space Shuttle Disaster
Scleroderma	Snake Bite	Ect......................

The largest percentage of untimely deaths are due to a very small gang of diseases—each of which can now be identified earlier than ever with new technology. If we take advantage of this technology now, today, we can overcome the greatest threats to a long, healthy life.

Bad things do happen and everyone dies. Freak accidents, toxic shock, pancreatic cancer, unexpected asthma, Lou Gehrig's disease, all tragic causes of death—but for unavoidable reasons. What makes dying stupid is when it *could* have been avoided.

Academy Award winner George C. Scott, best known for his famous portrayal of General George Patton, died in 1999 of a ruptured aortic aneurysm. This is a defect that can be easily detected and repaired *before* it takes a life. An ultrasound machine screens for an enlarged area of the aorta with almost 100 percent accuracy.

I don't know the details, but I doubt Mr. Scott's perfectly competent physicians thought to look for an aneurysm as part of his plan of care. After all, have you and your physician ever discussed screening for an aneurysm? It's painless, harmless, and dirt cheap. There are a lot of aneurysms out there. Some are time bombs, and most can be defused. But if your physician is not aware of your risk or options, where does that leave you? I'd say that leaves you in the driver's seat; it is, after all, your life.

I'm not suggesting you obsess about your health—just the opposite. I want you to address it effectively once or twice a year and move on, secure in the knowledge that you are not slipping through the ever-expanding cracks in America's healthcare system.

The best that modern medicine has for keeping you alive and healthy is almost certainly not on the menu of your health benefits. I want you to know what's available and how to get it. Here, you will find practical information that is not complicated or time-consuming to put into action with the help of your physician.

I will focus on the big-ticket killers, the few diseases that are most likely to cut your life short. They have become too mundane to make the late night news, too ordinary to get the attention they deserve. This is not about scaring you. It's about empowering you.

Our life expectancy is 30 years longer than our great-grandparent's. We live in a country with the world's most advanced medical knowledge and technology. When they fall ill, people from all over the world flock to the United States to obtain the most effective treatments available. Something, then, is terribly wrong when millions are dying from preventable diseases when, in fact, their prevention is a straightforward and manageable process.

Why are we failing? It's not from a lack of desire, effort, or access to powerful medical tools, but from our human tendency to ignore "potential" problems plus our individual and collective investment in misinformed, wasted efforts.

Subtle traps lurk in human nature that lead both doctors and patients to bad choices. Decisions, made with the best of intentions and for all the right reasons, can and do kill. These medical "wrong turns" often stem from outdated belief systems, misleading information from the media, or from our amazing, but terribly flawed, healthcare system. In other words: *Bogus Beliefs*, *Bad Data* and a *Broken Bureaucracy*.

Bogus Beliefs

History is constantly rubbing our nose in the facts. When a long-held belief is completely disproved, convincing the public to change its collective mindset is a huge undertaking and usually requires a fall guy. Take poor Galileo. He was imprisoned for arguing that the sun, not the Earth, is the center of our solar system.

We all have a hard time letting go of what we've accepted to be true. We cling to the beliefs we acquired as children, even when faced with undeniable proof that they are false.

Usually, being wrong is no big deal. One can believe the earth is flat and go right on living. Being wrong about science and our health, on the other hand, can be fatal.

Madame Curie's pioneering work with radioactive elements like radium led to her fame and the honor of a Nobel Prize. It also caused the leukemia that killed her. Today, we recognize that radiation is nothing to play with. We *do* learn. We don't expose our kids to lead paint or second-hand smoke. We buckle our seat belts and, when

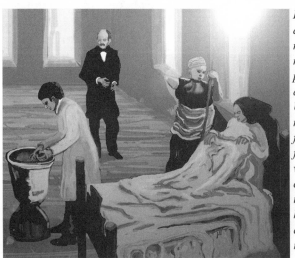

Dr. Ignaz Semmelweis discovered the primary reason for the extremely high maternal death rate 1847 and proved his theory in two different hospital settings. Unbelievably, his colleagues ridiculed and disregarded his findings. One simple, cost-free step could have saved the vast majority of lives lost after childbirth. History reveals that sometimes inertia in the healthcare community contributes to the stupid reasons people die.

necessary, get flu shots. We know how to run away from danger.

Unfortunately, we don't move so fast to eliminate threats of a different kind. I'm talking about our failure to quickly implement life-saving discoveries. When a new way to prolong life or prevent disease is discovered, it is often either rejected or treated apathetically for years before its benefits become widely accepted.

Consider this: In the 1840s, 30 years before Louie Pasteur developed his "germ theory" of disease, 20 percent of new mothers in the hospitals of Vienna, Austria died a few days after giving birth. The cause, "childbed fever," was three times more common in hospital deliveries than in women giving birth with midwives. Yet Vienna physician, Ignaz Semmelweis, had clearly demonstrated an astounding drop in the maternal death rate of hospital deliveries, down to less than 1 percent of mothers, simply by requiring one thing of his staff: that they wash their hands with water and a bit of chlorine.

Hand washing brought the safety of giving birth to an unprecedented level, possibly the lowest maternal death rate that human childbirth had yet seen. Dr. Semmelweis pleaded with the other doctors and students to do the same, especially after coming from their autopsy class, before delivering babies.

Yet his message was ignored and often disdained by his colleagues. After all, they "knew" disease came from an imbalance of the body's four humours, not dirty hands. In frustration, Dr. Semmelweis resigned and moved to another maternity clinic. There, he showed the same benefits from hand washing, an admittedly inconvenient practice at the time, but again faced ridicule and scorn. Even after his death, he was the object of derision in his field.

Ignaz Philipp Semmelweis 1818 - 1865

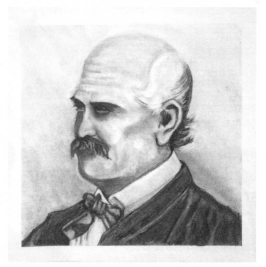

Doing things "the way they were always done" cost the lives of countless new mothers even when the facts about infection were undeniable. Decades passed before hand washing became the standard of care in medicine. Clearly, our natural resistance to change can cost society dearly.

So can language. This essential tool is a double-edged sword. Humans are unique in how we use language to communicate, understand our world, organize, categorize, and share experiences.

But in the process, we attach emotion to words in ways that attract or repel us. We back away from suggestions of pain or fear. We race toward what we interpret as pleasure, comfort, and security. These categorizations help keep us from harm. Would anyone you know touch the pretty blue flame on a stove more than once?

Unfortunately, the emotions we attach to words do not always serve us well. Many people associate medicine with poison, chemical, or something artificial. They may also believe any food or remedy labeled "All Natural" is good for their health. The fact is, *natural* has very little to do with better health, and sometimes a *chemical* isn't half bad.

"Drug" is another emotionally charged label. What is a drug, anyway? Is a woman on estrogen therapy taking a drug or a natural substance that replaces what she's lost? Music alters one's mental state. Does that make it a drug? What makes a drug "good" or "bad"? We will explore these issues and examine widespread prejudices and misconceptions, exposing how our views become distorted, with serious consequences for our health and well-being.

Bad Data

Information that *seems* to make sense influences our opinions and decisions but may be only partly accurate or incomplete. The military knows all too well that almost, but not totally accurate information is usually much more dangerous than *no* information.

Every day, we are at the mercy of an avalanche of external and internal messages. The information we act upon, *often inaccurate*, comes from the outside world—the media, the government, advertisers, the Internet, friends and family. Errors also originate from within the fascinating workings of our own human minds.

Most of us, while intelligent and educated, operate from an incomplete understanding of how medical knowledge actually becomes *known*. This is different from just being wrong. It amounts to taking accurate information, processing it through our individual mental and emotional software to come up with skewed interpretations and incorrect conclusions.

Health information is uniquely susceptible to distortion by this usually reliable process. The way we naturally think and the way most medical information is organized DO NOT MATCH. Medical facts exist mostly in *statistical* form and only have meaning when they are interpreted and applied in this form. It's all about probabilities.

For example, *statistically*, a popular blood pressure medicine may carry a risk of serious kidney damage. An alarmed patient, hearing this report on the evening news, tosses his bottle of the drug into the garbage. What he is missing is that the risk only applies to patients with a specific medical condition, something his doctor *knows* he does not have. For most people, the kidney risk does not exist at all, while taking the medicine can mean a substantially longer life. Heard the right story—got the wrong message. On the other hand, the newest life-saving miracle cholesterol drug might be worthless for certain patients, offer no benefit at all, and put them at needless risk for side-effects.

Anyone can learn what statistical information on a subject means *for them*, but it doesn't come naturally. Our minds decipher information in terms of cause and effect, filtering everything new through our past experiences. Our emotionally colored "this-means-that" way of interpreting the world serves us well in many cases, but it is a huge disadvantage when trying to apply scientific findings to our individual situation.

Let's face it, if everyone made choices independent of emotions like greed, fear, or lust, and became instinctively good at probability and statistics, every casino in the world would close overnight. Don't hold your breath.

The news media and advertising industry, fully aware of how we respond to new information, give us brief, intriguing, and oversimplified sound bytes to get the results they're looking for: high ratings or big sales. Even if you're blessed (or cursed) with a statistical mind, you must go beyond the hype and the partial, condensed reporting to get the facts that affect you personally.

This wouldn't be a big deal if the worst that happened were unnecessary purchases due to slick advertising. But when it comes to your health, reacting to misleading information is dangerous.

Fortunately, we can train our minds to use the best available information in the most useful way. It involves asking a few simple questions whenever you hear an alarming news report about a medication or other health issue.

Let's say the news of the day is, "Woman dies after taking an anti-depressant." Before flushing away an effective medication or lining up for the class-action lawsuit, an alarmed viewer, taking the same medication, might ask:

> ▶ **Is there evidence her death was *directly* caused by the drug, or were other medical conditions or emotional problems the cause?**

> ▶ **How many similar patients might commit suicide because they are *not* on this medication?**

> ▶ **What are the risks to me of stopping this medicine, especially if I do it abruptly?**

The answers to simple questions like these help clear away the confusion for patients who hear something scary about medication or a medical procedure.

A heartfelt warning: Never stop taking a prescribed medication because of something you hear or read *until* you talk to your doctor.

Broken Bureaucracy

Again, people who can afford it come from all over the world to take advantage of our country's medical services—and for good reason! Medical miracles are performed more often in the U.S. than anywhere else. Yet our healthcare system is also the party most responsible for the failure to prevent unnecessary death. It's a safety net with gaping holes.

Despite criticisms I offer in this book, I wouldn't trade the quality and content of medical care in the United States for any other in the world. But why does our healthcare system fail to stop diseases that are, in fact, stoppable?

Because our healthcare system reflects our human nature: we react to a disaster *after* it happens far better than we anticipate and act upon an impending crisis. Experts and government officials *knew* a major hurricane in New Orleans was likely and would be devastating. Yet the necessary preventive measures were not taken. We are now paying the price for a predictable catastrophe in terms of lost, uprooted families, destroyed property, the long-term impact on a unique culture, and billions of taxpayer dollars. New Orleans will never be the same.

That directly parallels our healthcare system. It is absolutely clear what can be done to save tens of thousands of lives every year. We just don't do it.

Consider our major killers: heart disease, stroke, and cancer. We don't practice the very best medicine, the "state of the art," when it comes to preventing these diseases or screening to find them in time to disarm them. Instead, physicians are *encouraged* to practice what's called the "standard of care," a level of care based on information that is typically five to ten years out of date. Medical science moves extremely fast, and this creates an enormous gap in quality between providing the *status quo* and providing the best available care in preventing disease.

Most patients and many doctors are not aware the gap exists. Why? Many factors influence how physicians practice, but high on the list of barriers is this: patients *and* physicians have bought into a system where the insurance industry dictates what physicians "can" and "can't" do. Control has been turned over to entities that have a glaring conflict of interest.

They are measured first and foremost by their profits or, for government-funded programs, by how well they manage money. They are not measured by the success of their policies in preserving health and life. They choose the care they will "cover" based on how little it costs to provide what is considered "standard." Insurers rigorously resist paying for new tests, procedures, and treatments for as long as possible, even if they are a major improvement over current standards. The widespread use of medical advancements can be stalled for decades—yes, decades—based on the industry's arbitrary claim that they are still "experimental."

I'm not suggesting there is a conspiracy against patients by the medical community or insurance industry. They are victims as well, victims of a healthcare system that has taken on a life of its own that limits and disables the content and scope of our preventive medical care.

Remember the response when Dr. Semmelweis demonstrated to his colleagues that clean hands save lives? Thousands more women died needlessly, because no one wanted to change the standard of care. How can patients advocate for their own healthcare if physicians are pressured to maintain, or voluntarily cling to, the *status quo*?

Intellectual inertia is part of human nature, but the world of medicine carries the consequences to a new level. Combined with the financial interests of government and insurance agencies and with our own passivity as patients, we have created a "perfect storm" for failure.

Now, back to you, the individual. As long as you rely on someone else to ensure you get the care you think you deserve and to pay the entire bill on your behalf, you will wind up with the *least* that modern medicine is willing to offer. Not because healthcare providers don't want you to have the best, but because our healthcare system can barely afford your annual check-up.

If you want the best modern medicine has to give, it's going to take a little time and money—yours. It will also require you to have some fresh insights and solid facts to enable you to be your own best advocate. Ready to start?

BOGUS BELIEFS

*"Words, thoughts, and mental images directly affect our moods and the reactions of our bodies. The words we choose **matter**."*

Chapter 2

What's in a Name?

Shakespeare's Romeo mused, "That which we call a rose by any other name would smell as sweet." But would it?

Romeo's family name, Montague, and that of Juliet, Capulet, sparked such violent prejudice between their families that the young lovers were destroyed by the conflict.

Like many creatures, humans communicate with gestures, non-verbal body language, facial expressions, and grunts. But we came to dominate this planet, because we also communicate with each other using language. We *name* things.

Our use of language is anything but simple. "Capulet" did more than identify a family member. It conjured up feelings of hatred and fear to every member of the Montague family, and vice versa.

Names wield power. Beyond a mere label, each one gets filtered through our knowledge, experiences, and beliefs, sometimes provoking strong emotions and often altering the word's original meaning.

"Murder" and "suffocate" are just verbs that describe actions, but they also creep me out. Just hearing and typing them drains my energy. By contrast, my spirits are lifted at the mention of "coffee" or "vacation."

And I'm not just imagining it. Progress in psychology and neuroscience has begun to demystify the workings of the human mind. Words, thoughts, and mental images directly affect our moods and the reactions of our bodies. The words we choose *matter*. They influence our thoughts and feelings and the other choices we make, including those about our own health.

How do you react when you hear the word "disease"? What images appear in your mind's eye? What are you feeling?

I picture old *LIFE* magazine photographs of famine, filth, death and suffering, along with a few scary dermatology photographs that both frightened and fascinated me as a kid.

How about the word "healthy"? I see children at play, happy dogs with shining fur, lush green trees with perfectly ripe fruit, and active people enjoying friends and their highly functional families. I feel physically better thinking about "health" than "disease." Who wouldn't?

What is "disease"? Is it anything short of perfect health? For that matter, is there any such thing as perfect health, especially as we age?

Some people believe that every trial or tribulation, every unhealthy or destructive behavior, every situation that causes physical or emotional distress is a disease, and they want a validating medical description and 100 percent insurance coverage to return things to "normal."

This attitude distances the person from their problem. The problem becomes an external force, an outside evil that is victimizing them. It relieves them from their part in the problem *and* from paying for treatment. If this thinking was universal, we'd all take the role of helpless victim, assuming some mystical entity would accept the responsibility and cost for making us all better.

On the other hand, for some people there is no such thing as a disease. Who are we to mess around with Mother Nature? Sure, a little boy with sickle cell anemia may die painfully after years of suffering from his inherited genetic condition, but they know sickle cell is a *natural* result of a perfectly *natural* mutation caused by a perfectly *natural* process of evolutionary forces.

This is true, but disavowing sickle cell anemia does not end the suffering. Instead, it undermines efforts to alter these "natural" occurrences to save or improve young lives.

Both ways of looking at disease are dangerous because they are extreme, but the absurdities we find in these examples are often evident in our general notions of health and illness. Labeling a condition a "disease" gives it validity that often commands sympathy and insurance dollars. When science and economics cross paths, debates rage over where healthcare dollars are spent and which medical research should be funded. Observing this process will influence our opinions and expectations about our healthcare.

Is alcoholism truly a disease? What about Attention Deficit Hyperactivity Disorder (ADHD)? Or, are they just a way of making "self-destructive drunks" and "lazy parents" feel better about themselves? Can *all* self-destructive behaviors be classified as diseases?

These classifications, "official disease" or not, determine how much money will be spent on each problem and *who* will have to do the spending. To decision makers at insurance companies and policy makers in government, labels of this sort directly influence the content and availability of the healthcare services they must offer. So they must try to influence our expectations by "spinning" the popular language we use about each issue.

What about you? Do these classifications help or can they hinder your attempts to improve and prolong your life and the lives of your loved ones?

Once we attach a name to a medical condition, our subconscious mind doesn't separate the title from all its subjective baggage. Many people believe that a child labeled with Attention Deficit Hyperactivity Disorder actually has a *deficit* and is *disordered.* The facts prove otherwise. Many children labeled as ADHD have above average IQs.

Then again, many of them fail in school, develop addictions, or end up in jail. Perhaps they grew up being *treated* as deficient, disorderly, damaged individuals.

Doctors, like everyone else, use labels to communicate with patients. Many medical terms become popular buzz words like "good cholesterol" or "flesh-eating bacteria." Colorful language, but inaccurate. Patients interpret words like these through their individual emotional filters before they communicate with family and friends. They internalize and share *their interpretation* of what the doctor said. Some will also incorporate whatever they find on Google into that interpretation and wind up with a message completely different from what the doctor intended to communicate. Ever play the game of "telephone" as a child? Same result—a lot of nonsense at the other end of the line.

Assigning a name to a condition can certainly be comforting. We breathe a sigh of relief that the problem isn't imagined. A name validates it as something real, specific and, hopefully, treatable. We feel less vulnerable because the unknown is now known. But feelings of control achieved only through the naming process are make-believe.

"I have fibromyalgia; that's why I hurt all the time."

"I have Epstein-Barr; that's why I have no energy to do anything."

The pain and fatigue are real. The names may not be. The labels for chronic pain or fatigue have changed from decade to decade, and yet the misery these patients suffer has been around for centuries. Physicians are no longer convinced that chronic muscle pain and profound fatigue are due to an imbalance of the four bodily humours or caused by demonic possession. Fifty years from now, they won't be called Fibromyalgia or Epstein-Barr syndrome.

Clinging to a title that makes their disease "official" may actually prevent a patient from utilizing therapies that may help them. A patient may refuse to consider a treatment used for disorders of mood or of a dysfunctional sleeping pattern, because it is inconsistent with his "diagnosis."

Of course, assigning a name to something and putting it in a category provides a *starting place* for discussion and understanding. From there, however, it's easy to stray from the facts into assumptions. Our minds *want* to pigeonhole everything. It's our nature. Someone says *cancer.* People gasp. Their minds immediately file it under *suffering and death*. Yet, if you looked beyond that first reaction at the facts and details about the conditions, I'm pretty sure I could talk you into choosing prostate cancer for yourself or your spouse over sugar diabetes any day of the week.

Let's get away from relying on a name to make us feel informed. We need to go deeper, expand our understanding about what is actually known and what is still unknown about any condition. This enables us to avoid prepackaged half-truths or incorrect beliefs that are so easily attached to a label.

Is alcoholism a disease or not? ***Who cares?*** It is something that destroys health, human potential, and families. The questions that need to be answered are: What can be done to improve the life and health of the person abusing alcohol? What do we do when someone's abuse of alcohol is a threat to others? What do we know or need to find out about alcoholism that leads to effective treatment?

What about Ritalin? Is it a way to eliminate some "deficit" in children labeled as ADHD? Or does it correct a "chemical imbalance"? Is it possible these children would have been considered completely normal according to society's standards a few hundred years ago? Is it possible these wonderful children simply do not fit easily into this modern, artificially-created information age? If so, maybe it's our society that is diseased.

Tom Cruise and many others may claim that treating such a child with medication is a copout, the expedient use of a toxic chemical that could destroy their personalities. Could medication also be an effective way for a child to develop and perform more in the mainstream of society, at a stage of life where being "in the mainstream" is critical to his or her self-esteem and future success? We should focus on questions like these when trying to address the needs of a child struggling at home or in school, not whether or not little Johnny is actually *in* or *out* of the ADHD club.

What about depression? Bad attitude or helpless victim of disease? How about skin color? Would Snow White be considered diseased if she washed up on a shadeless desert island where none of the dark-skinned natives wore clothes? She'd spend most of her life painfully sunburned, while the natives of the island did just fine. Would she be suffering from *skin-pigment-deficit-disorder*? Again, it doesn't matter how you label Ms. White's skin situation; what matters is to understand it, and doing what we can to improve her life.

Are high blood pressure and high cholesterol the natural consequences of being a couch potato, or are they diseases in their own right? Are patients with these conditions *defective*? If so, a lot of defective humans are running this country, our corporations, military, churches, universities, and police departments. By the way, just a few years ago their numbers doubled almost overnight.

People didn't change, only our words did. In September 2002, the National Cholesterol Education Program (NCEP) an authority that publishes guidelines for doctors to use in the treatment of high cholesterol, once again lowered the cholesterol level that it considers to be acceptable.

In May 2003, the Joint National Committee on Prevention (JNC) did the same for acceptable levels of blood pressure. These changes meant that millions of people, whose cholesterol or blood pressure had been considered normal, now found themselves in the abnormal category. They went to bed "healthy" and woke up "diseased."

Emotionally, we withdraw from concepts that we consider upsetting. This detachment gets in the way of understanding and addressing problems that affect our health and well-being. If we don't think about it, it might go away. Men are the worst. I know. I'm one of them. We instinctively deny any health problem because that would suggest we are "weak" or "abnormal" or "girly men." Subconsciously, we attach a negative self-image to words like "disease" or "disorder." Yet we don't necessarily consider other men weak or abnormal because they have high blood pressure —after all, *they're* only human.

I can usually identify the exact second a patient stops listening. The mind freezes and then the facial expression. He tunes me out and ups the volume on his inner voice: *"Huh? Me? No way! I've never felt better! Gotta cut this short. Things to do, people to see. Hell, doctors* **have** *to find something wrong, that's how they make the big bucks..."*

I estimate about half my patients have a fundamental discomfort with the idea of taking medication, any medication. They tell me they just don't take pills, not even aspirin for a headache.

For many, taking a drug is like surrendering to decay and death. It implies they are turning into grandma or grandpa whose final chapter was so pathetic, their frail bodies useless as they swallowed one pill after another.

Some patients are opposed to taking medicine, because manifesting a condition like high blood pressure, diabetes, depression, etc., makes them feel like failures. Redemption can only come if they fix the condition through strength of character.

Unless doctors have the time and expertise to provide psychotherapy as well as medical care, they can't adequately address misconceptions like these. Often the result is that patients let their emotions, not reason, guide their response to a health issue. They reject a simple preventive measure, such as taking a new medication or undergoing a non-standard screening test, and as a result may live shorter lives.

The emotional connection between accepting medical treatment and surrendering to disease is deeply rooted in our culture, in part, because of the history of medical treatment itself. Only a few decades ago, there were few drugs that *prevented* disease. Drug therapy was used only after someone became seriously ill, too late in many cases for a cure. A visit by the doctor rarely did much to change the outcome of the disease, so his presence came to signify that death was approaching.

Today, with the vast array of medications that can and should be prescribed to prevent rather than treat serious conditions, our cultural mindset is still stuck on the concept of using drugs to treat disease instead of preventing healthy people from becoming sick. Doctors are part of the same culture and subconsciously err on the side of *under*-treating the risks for heart attacks, strokes, and cancer. The patient is delighted. *No drugs! I'm f-i-n-e! Death is not waiting in the wings!*

Consider Bob. He doesn't want to take the blood pressure drug his doctor recommends. Doc, also prone to perceptions from the past, doesn't relish the possibility of causing Bob some annoying side-effect or extra expense—not to mention making him feel, you know, less like a man. So Doc is willing to give it a few more months—the "wait and watch" approach. He'll give Bob an opportunity to get his blood pressure under control on his own. And Bob is determined to start immediately on an exercise program and to give up his favorite desserts.

Months have somehow turned into years. Doc certainly didn't have the time or resources to follow along behind Bob to see how he managed his own health regimen. Meanwhile, after his initial passionate commitment, Bob got distracted by life. With no success in losing weight or becoming the athlete he envisioned, he avoids the unpleasant prospect of returning to his doctor as the failure he sees himself to be. This is how we lose a lot of Bobs. Sooner instead of later.

You're a rational person. Feeling ashamed or flawed or vulnerable is the exact *opposite* of how you should feel when taking a necessary, properly prescribed medication. Discussing the pros and cons, risks and benefits of taking a medicine intended to prolong your life should have you walking out of your doctor's office proud that you are participating in determining your fate based on reason, not fear.

We are each dealt a hand of biological cards. We decide what to do with them. I was born with extreme myopia, near-sightedness. I choose to wear corrective lenses instead of walking around looking "cool" until I collide with something. No one faults me for that decision. No one suggests I'm less of a man. I was also born with high cholesterol. I choose to lower it with a drug. Unlike wearing glasses, however, millions of people would *not* make that choice.

The cholesterol issue seems quite different. It's more abstract; it doesn't affect my day-to-day functioning as would near-blindness. Conceivably, the lowering of my cholesterol could be achieved through a low-fat diet and aerobic exercise. But I've chosen an expedient path to lower my cholesterol, apparently unwilling to step up to the plate, accept the cards I was dealt, and jog or diet my way to good health.

We all know this, and it colors our opinion of someone who chooses to take a drug for the same purpose.

Yet, the two decisions, wearing glasses and taking medication, are essentially the same. In both cases, the problems are genetic and, if ignored, can hurt me. And, in each case, the problem is *most effectively* resolved with a prescription.

You might not agree with my decision. Perhaps you've been alarmed by a tele-medical "expert" who lectures on the dangers of *toxic* drugs. He may even want them all pulled from the market. Why not choose *his* diet and purchase his all-natural supplements instead?

Most of us will decide based on how we *feel* instead of what we *know* or should know about the facts. We start forming ideas of good and bad, right and wrong, normal and abnormal, as kids. Our parents are usually our first and strongest influence. Then, through observation and trial and error, we figure out what the outside world—friends, teachers, coaches, someone else's parents, and cultural heroes—considers acceptable. We revise certain opinions to fit into our world. We also learn which beliefs and actions are downright dangerous to express or defend. After all, we don't want to be labeled "freaks."

Our belief system literally becomes part of us, forming permanent patterns in our brains. It "burns in" our emotional and cognitive attitudes about the world at large, the people in our lives, new information, and the words that define all of those things.

Weird, isn't it, that our feelings and opinions can be etched into our brains like a computer program onto a silicon chip? But they are, and they're very difficult to rewrite. Why else would so many unfounded prejudices and superstitions remain powerful, long after our society's so-called enlightenment?

Hard-wired opinions of what's good-for-me versus what's bad-for-me play out in everyone's medical decisions. All of us, including healthcare providers, are deeply attached to certain beliefs about health that can make us blind even to overwhelming evidence if it's contrary to our beliefs.

I remember a 1960s TV program, *You Asked For It*, in which a reporter asked Texans to name the largest state in the Union. Many insisted it was Texas. Honest mistake. Alaska hadn't been a state all that long. But even after the interviewer provided geographical proof that Alaska was much larger, some Texans still refused to accept the facts. One actually suggested that he and the reporter duke it out. To him, Texas will always be the largest state in Union.

Sometimes ignoring the facts isn't a big deal. There's no harm if a Texan chooses to believe his state is bigger than Alaska. But fiercely protected beliefs do not change reality. And sometimes it *is* a big deal. The conviction that you can outmaneuver genetically-high cholesterol with a daily run can be a fatal mistake.

When it comes to health risks, substituting a delusional idea for sound scientific reasoning may help you *feel* in control of your destiny—right up to the moment your heart seizes. Of course, exercise and a reasonable diet are important to overall health and longevity. But these things alone do not diffuse nature's time bombs. In many cases, the right medication will.

In taking action to lower cholesterol, is it really the cholesterol number that matters? Getting a lower cholesterol score may turn out to be part of our plan, but isn't our *goal* to avoid a heart attack or a stroke? Seems obvious? Maybe.

But considering the number of young people who die this way, it's safe to say we're losing sight of that goal. It is the artery-hardening process itself, not a cholesterol level in the blood that can destroy the heart. So the goal is to stop that process in time.

The same logic applies to measurements of blood pressure, blood sugar, and many of the other "scores" we like to collect. I shouldn't care whether the numbers look good on paper. I want to do what it takes to prevent that heart attack, that stroke, or some other needless disaster.

How did cholesterol get to be center stage in the national campaign to prevent heart attacks and strokes? In health and medicine, history plays a large part in determining how we behave. Back in the '60s, researchers noticed that groups of people with higher cholesterol had more heart attacks and strokes than average. At that time, there was no effective medication to lower cholesterol, so researchers tried to identify foods high in cholesterol. They hoped that giving the public a list of foods to avoid would lead to fewer heart attacks and strokes. Goodbye, eggs, red meat and butter.

The fallout from that era is that eggs still have a bad rap, even though it turns out they're *not* bad for you. Somehow, the part that really matters —the not dying part—got lost in the national focus on our cholesterol scoreboard.

Doctors aren't immune to this. We often pay more attention to getting the number right while overlooking the fact that *how* we treat cholesterol, and how we alter the size and chemistry of the tiny particles that carry it in our blood, is as important to our patients' survival as getting them a passing grade on their cholesterol blood test.

Here's the thing. The majority of people who suffer heart attacks in this country actually have *normal cholesterol levels,* sometimes quite low. This is a statistical fact. Yes, scientists found that people with high cholesterol have an above-average risk for a heart attack, but what the media failed to understand and communicate, and what the general public still doesn't realize is that the average chance of a heart attack is already really high, and normal cholesterol levels *do not* give us some kind of free pass. High cholesterol just makes an existing risk even greater.

Most people who work faithfully to lower their cholesterol through low-fat diets don't necessarily live any longer or have fewer heart attacks than those who do nothing to change their levels. Most people who adhere to their low-fat, low-cholesterol diet and rigorous exercise schedule will lower their cholesterol a maximum of 10 percent to 15 percent. That translates into only a 3 percent to 5 percent reduction in their chance of dying young.

All that work for so little improvement in life expectancy.

Here was my personal decision-making process. Either I had to try lowering my cholesterol level through diet, exercise, and a vitamin-packed lifestyle, or I had to take medication.

I elected to take a medication that lowers my cholesterol levels up to 60 percent—four times more than the most extreme diets—but, more important, the pill has been shown time and again to lower the risk of a heart attack or stroke by 22 percent to 65 percent. Low-fat diet and exercise have not.

The pill I take doubles my chances of being around to see my grandchildren grow up. Actually, right now I do it all. I take the medication, eat a reasonable diet, and I exercise—not fanatically but regularly. I do it all because it makes me feel better physically, but I know which one of these actions is doing the most for my heart.

If I chose to forego the medication and to eat only foods labeled "healthy" while running five miles every day, I might be viewed by others with admiration for my willpower and stamina, for taking matters into my own hands like a real man. I'd also be increasing the chance of leaving my wife and kids without a husband and father. Some hero.

There are thousands of books, magazines, and TV programs repeating the same standard messages about diet and exercise. The biggest impact they seem to have is to leave the public limp with guilt.

These messages simply stress "good clean living" as the secret to glowing health and longevity. Most of us, living busy, complex, and stressful 21st century lives, don't find it easy to maintain a daily regimen of an ideal diet-exercise program. When we don't "measure up," we feel like failures. Then, when success seems beyond our reach, we give up the game altogether.

For millions of people like me, born with high cholesterol, a rigorous diet and exercise program alone are not enough to reduce the risk of a heart attack. What can make the difference is a drug.

All the fruits, vegetables, and vitamin supplements in the world won't prevent most cancer deaths. What can make the difference is simple screening that can detect cancer in time to stop it in its tracks.

Our words generate feelings. And feelings can get in the way of facts. If we gravitate exclusively toward the words, subjects, and ideas that feel warm and nurturing, and ignore those we've learned to react to with suspicion or discomfort, we close the door on a world of life-saving possibilities.

The answer is balance. Realistic goals for diet, exercise, and lifestyle do matter, but it can be a fatal mistake to think they are all that are needed to prevent a life-threatening disease.

Now, I'd like to introduce you to my nemesis. She is a major reason I'm writing this book. She's been worshiped, adored, revered, and feared since the beginning of mankind, but she has absolutely no conscience. No compassion.

Many people are fooled by her breathtaking beauty. It's easy to miss what motivates her—a cruel, callous, and calculating indifference. She is a force you do not want to underestimate.

*"There is no universal good or bad, right or wrong,
healthy or unhealthy about the 'naturalness' of a substance.
Echinacea is a natural substance. So is penicillin. So is cyanide."*

Chapter 3

Sorry, Mother Doesn't Care if You Live or Die

You know what it takes to live a long, happy life. Escape our high-pressure, emotionally-charged, crazy-making culture and get in tune with nature. *Mother* Nature. Live in harmony with her beauty and bounty. Let her nurture, heal, sustain, protect, and renew your soul.

Mother has been revered by all civilizations that recognize how human survival relies on her good graces. Our modern, enlightened, high-tech society still believes, as nomadic tribes did, that Mother Nature exists to keep us alive and well. So we bow to her wisdom and gentle harmonious teachings. When we step out the door into a glorious, serene spring morning, well, who could argue with her beauty or power?

Mother *is* the source of everything we need to exist: air, water, food, wind, and fire. She deserves to be appreciated and respected.

But not trusted.

She has a dark side. I don't just mean flood, famine, pestilence, and earthquakes. I mean damaged genes, the plague, unfathomable pain, disability, death by, uh, *natural* causes.

My family loves the wilderness that surrounds our community. The Cascade mountain range, roaring rivers, serene lakes, open meadows and forests. It's easy to drop my guard as I admire nature in all her glory on a Saturday morning hike. But I'm in the guarding business, and, when my first patient Monday morning is a patient with cerebral palsy or diabetic blindness, I must deal with Mother on an entirely different level. I face the grim reality that her interest in these people is merely one of curiosity, not compassion.

Life on planet Earth has been evolving and shifting over billions of years. Only recently have humans begun adapting nature to our needs, effectively accelerating this process. We began to alter the natural plant life with farming and the natural animal life with domestic livestock. Fruit trees, vegetables, and grains produce more food per plant than their recent ancestors, and the docile cattle, sheep, and chickens of today are known to bear little resemblance to their more aggressive ancestors of just a few thousand years ago.

It's tempting to believe that these necessities of life were put here *deliberately* for our benefit. But in fact, just like the life forms we rely on for survival, we humans were shaped and culled and eventually became the creatures we are as a *response* to the environment. Nature is the cause; we are just one of her effects. Mother has always been a detached manipulator—playing with and experimenting on all forms of life. Ours included. And she does it on a grand scale.

Thomas Edison stated he learned a thousand ways *not* to make a light bulb before finally discovering how to transform electricity into light. His trials and errors were nothing compared to Mother's experiments. Edison focused and directed his work with a *deliberate* goal in mind, yet he still suffered a thousand defeats for one success. By contrast, Nature's fiddling around is completely random, occasionally striking pay dirt, like the opposable thumb, but hitting dead ends, literally, millions of times more often.

The forces of Nature mutate life, a little at a time, often invisible to the naked eye. They cause genetic changes through radiation, DNA transcription errors and other mechanisms that alter the existing code. Organism by organism, she plays around to see what turns up. The great experiment goes on, advancing certain members of a species a tiny bit at a time while, at the same time and through the same processes, hurting or killing millions more along the way.

Sickle Cell Anemia is a simple but elegant example of both effects.

This single mutation in the genetic code for hemoglobin, found mostly in people of African descent, is harmless to children unless both parents pass on the defective form of the gene to their child. In that case, the child's abnormal hemoglobin molecules can stack together in his red blood cells to form long, rigid structures, morphing the cells from smooth disks into sharp, pointed sickle shapes.

These cells plug up capillaries, and the result is a sickle cell crisis, an excruciating event that can last days or weeks and wreak havoc on oxygen-starved organs. The crisis is a living hell for the child and for the family at the bedside. The life span of such children, while improving slowly with research, is seriously reduced, and the quality of life pretty grim.

Yet, the sickle cell mutation is believed to be a *benefit* to the individual who inherits the defective gene from *only one* parent, because it provides some protection against deadly malaria. In Africa, that is a very good thing. In the United States, it is neither good nor bad. And, for a child *anywhere* who inherits the defective gene from both parents, it is a tragedy.

If you've ever sat with such a person during a crisis, it is easy to view Mother Nature as the enemy. However, she's neither an ally nor a predator. She isn't intentionally out to get us, and she isn't here to save us. Whether we live or die, individually or as an entire civilization, is of no interest to her.

We're here because our species hasn't yet been wiped out by her ongoing experiments, and because we haven't yet done ourselves in. This is *our* time on the planet. Keep in mind, however, that for every species alive today, thousands are now extinct.

I've never heard it better said than by author, Sam Harris:

> The very mechanisms that create the incredible beauty and diversity of the living world guarantee monstrosity and death. The child born without limbs, the sightless fly, the vanished species—these are nothing less than Mother Nature caught in the act of throwing her clay.[1]

Brutality, violence, pain, and grief are not the monopoly of man and his inhumanity to man. They're an integral part of all life on earth. If you're a parent, imagine losing half of your children before their fifth birthday. I often think I might not survive such a loss, yet mankind has lived with this pain since prehistoric times.

Only in the last few hundred years have life expectancy and child mortality rates improved significantly, and nature had nothing to do with it. We have, in fact, needed to battle her greatest assassin—infection. Our species came up with the four greatest life-saving inventions of all time: soap, sewers, antibiotics, and vaccines. Of course, the brains brilliant enough to stop the spread of infection were her creation too. But it's up to us as individuals to use them for our own protection.

And, if nature can be a cold-hearted and indifferent mother, she's even worse after you've reached middle age. Now she's really no longer on our side! The strength of youth can allow some remarkable recoveries from illness and injury, but once we've past our reproductive years, our resistance to the harsh elements seems to evaporate as if dear old mom is done with us. I was born. I grew up. I've reproduced, thank you very much, and now she doesn't need me any more. And she really doesn't owe me a darn thing. The next generation is in place, and the species goes on. The rest of my life doesn't matter one bit to her. Nor should it. But it does to me.

One hundred years ago, our average life span was about 40 years. Imagine: infancy, childhood, 10 or 20 years of adulthood, death. We've always wanted more and have been willing to work for it.

Each generation has used their brains, creativity, and new scientific knowledge to buy more time. Today, most Americans can expect to live long enough to see their children grow up and to be part of their grandchildren's lives. But not because Mother Nature warmed up to us. She still doesn't care if we're around once our ability to procreate ends.

If we'd like long, healthy lives, we have to do it for ourselves. It's not on Mother's agenda. This means we have to take full control of our health. It means we have to make informed medical decisions and smarter lifestyle choices. We have to override mental programming formed by superstitious beliefs, obsolete information, and Madison Avenue hype. Here's one example that combines all three:

One hundred percent All Natural!

If I offer patients a choice between a supposedly natural versus artificial remedy, no matter the age, education, or IQ of the person I ask, the hands-down winner is: *Natural, doc.* When I ask how they define a natural treatment, the responses become vague, uncertain, posed more as a question. *Pure? No chemicals? Organic? Not toxic? No chemicals?*

Many people have a positive feeling about a product they buy in health food stores or naturopathic, chiropractic, and acupuncture clinics. They believe it is "of the earth herself" infused with an almost magical healing energy that is pure, safe, and wholesome, so long as it hasn't been touched by researchers, scientists, and quality control experts.

Early societies, you know, the ones where the life span was half of what it is today, had nothing *but* natural. They did their best with what Mother Nature had to offer.

Today, we have the wonders of mass marketing promoting a huge industry of natural anything, natural everything. The ad wizards know how the public feels about any product—food, remedies, vitamins, toothpaste, etc.—labeled natural. And they know the public is suspicious of products without that label: Probably unsafe. Probably a money-making, cancer-causing scam of evil corporations. It's all about emotion, not facts.

Natural. The word has been perverted, exploited, and shoved down our throats to sell everything from toilet paper to motor oil. So it might be in our best interest to know its definition. Here's the meaning as defined by *The Oxford American Dictionary*:

> **natural** (nach-u-ral) adj. 1. of, or existing in, or produced by nature.

That seems simple enough. Let's take a few examples: Tulips and butterflies in spring. A young mother beginning labor. A native boy climbing trees and splashing in the water. Each of these describes a scene easily found in nature before cities, cars, drugs, and pollution.

Now, look closer.

A tulip eaten by a young deer and a butterfly eaten by a bird. A young mother hemorrhaging to death during labor and delivery, leaving behind a doomed newborn. A young boy dying of lockjaw from a tiny splinter. A life expectancy of 32 years, and a 30 percent infant mortality rate. All common scenes found in nature before cities, cars, drugs, and pollution. Sometimes "All Natural" isn't all that pretty.

Yet every day we are hit with advertising claims of "All Natural," as though no other quality should be necessary to compel us to buy their amazing new product.

One day, I counted all the advertising messages I encountered for "All Natural" products—forty-three. Did you know there are "all natural" tampons and shaving creams? It was news to me. We all know that pharmaceutical "chemicals" in little pills are not natural, but maybe early man really could pick little time release gel caps off a melatonin tree to help him with his insomnia.

The concept of "natural medicine" is an oxymoron. Like any medical intervention, natural medicine involves a deliberate act, above and beyond nature. Concentrating any biologically active substance to swallow or apply to the body is not an act of nature but of man.

There is no universal good or bad, right or wrong, healthy or unhealthy about the "naturalness" of a substance. Echinacea is a natural substance. So is penicillin. So is cyanide.

It's perfectly natural for young people to get excited and make babies. That doesn't make it a good idea for a 14-year-old couple in today's society. It's natural for lightning to start a brushfire that clears debris from the forest floor, promoting new growth. It's not a good idea to let the fire rage on its own until it wipes out families and homes. Most of us would employ an unnatural water system to save our homes and our loved ones.

And yet, we may automatically reach for those "natural" products without a second thought other than the basic assumption it will be good for us. If, God forbid, it's a *chemical*, we are pretty sure it will slowly poison us, and we won't even know it until our hair falls out in clumps.

The only way to avoid being misled by your own beliefs and the effects of mass marketing is to become aware of them in the first place. If anything you come across claims to be natural, stop and ask yourself, "Does this occur in nature?" Shampoo with honey and milk added? Shaving cream? That multi-vitamin? Probably not.

But even if it does, ask yourself, "So what?" Does the fact that it's found in nature mean it's safer, more effective, and relevant to its application...to your life?

Let's look at the other side of the "natural" coin. *Artificial.* According to *The Oxford American Dictionary*:

> **artificial** (ahr-ti-fish-al) adj. 1. not originating naturally—made by human skill.

Here's my list: nuclear bombs; automatic weapons; cars emitting tons of CO_2; Twinkies; plastic everything; and the chlorofluorocarbons opening a hole in our planet's ozone shield—all artificial, man-made creations.

On the other side of my paper: vaccines that stop plagues like smallpox and polio; toilets that flush; antibiotics; sterilizing machines; surgical soap and instruments; a near-zero maternal death rate; a life expectancy of 80 years. None of these were gifts of nature.

I can hear you groaning, "Okay, I get the point!" But here are some artificial things in our lives that are often *touted* as natural by their advertisers: clothes; a chiropractic adjustment; acupuncture; bread; herbal and homeopathic medicines; soaps and moisturizing creams. These were either invented or artificially altered by man. They are about as natural as your toaster.

Our emotional reaction to the word "artificial" is also a conditioned response, not the result of conscious, informed thinking. You may equate the word "chemical" to "toxin," yet everything we are, every molecule that goes into the making of our bodies is a chemical. So are water, carbohydrates, vitamins, herbs, prescription medications, minerals, amino acids, and olive oil.

In the world of medicine, the word "artificial," like the word "natural," is not what makes something good or bad, healthy or toxic, safe or risky.

Our society has not yet developed a strong immunity to subtle marketing messages. Selling health food products is not just about promoting real, exaggerated, or bogus benefits. It's also about strong but subtle suggestions that all prescription medications are dangerous chemicals. We become conditioned to think we must avoid them or pay the price, and this affects our healthcare buying decisions, political views, even our moral opinions. We assume medication should only be a last resort.

Once you realize you may have idealized Mother Nature, you can appreciate her for what she is and accept what she is not. When I'm hiking with my family, I admire her for all the things she's done right. When I'm making a decision about my children's health, I am very aware of her dark side. She is an indiscriminate killer and an indifferent experimenter, a true sociopath, no more concerned about us as a species or as individuals than she was about the dinosaurs or the dodo bird.

I use the brain she gave me to understand she *does not love me*.

"Does this mean we are drugging our kids with a cupcake? You bet."

Chapter 4

Everyone's Addicted – Everything's a Drug

How can *everyone* be drug dependent? First, consider the word, "drug." In our national consciousness, it is associated with evil, poverty, despair, and death. Overdose. Addict. Domestic abuse. Whacked. Wasted.

What makes something a drug? Most people, for example, would say penicillin fits the description. It's a substance, totally foreign to the body, with potentially dangerous side-effects, deliberately taken for a medical purpose to fight dangerous infections. Heroin is a drug, again, foreign to the body and taken to feel un-naturally euphoric. So is cocaine. Marijuana. Prozac. Alcohol. Nicotine. Aspirin. Coffee—my personal drug of choice.

But do all drugs have to be *foreign* substances? Sometimes the line blurs between what is foreign and what is familiar to the chemistry of our bodies.

Narcotic pain killers, like codeine and morphine, are well known as addictive drugs. Both are foreign substances, and yet they copy the effects of the natural narcotics our bodies produce, endorphins. Your brain releases endorphins during times of injury or athletic stress. They cause a "runner's high," that great feeling you experience after a vigorous workout. They suppress excruciating pain if you are seriously injured, allowing you to deal with the situation.

Endorphins are the result of one of Mother's experiments on how man might, or might not, survive. It has been suggested that a major release of endorphins causes the elated feelings reported by those who had near-death experiences.

Physicians can't use endorphins as a pain medication because endorphins can't get to the brain from the bloodstream or stomach. They would need to be administered directly into the brain via needle or catheter in order to be effective. Man-made narcotics, the medicinal counterparts of endorphins, can be given orally or injected and will then cross the "blood-brain barrier" to act at the same sites as natural endorphins, sometimes much more effectively.

Okay, now what if real human endorphins *could* be administered into the body, cross the blood-brain barrier and provide sustained relief? It wouldn't be a "foreign" substance. It's a natural substance produced by the body. Would it be considered a drug?

Yes. It would be the *deliberate* use of the substance, *above and beyond natural levels produced by the body*, in order to have a deliberate effect. We'd feel less pain and have a narcotic "high."

Many of the drugs on the market actually *are* the same molecules the body manufactures: estrogen, insulin, human growth hormone, and tissue-plasminogen-activator used to save lives on the heels of a heart attack. Some are synthetic or animal-extracted mixtures, but many are 100 percent identical to the human form. One of the most abundant estrogens in the normal female body, 17-beta estradiol, is used as a treatment for menopause. Is it a drug?

Consider this situation: A 20-year-old woman must have her uterus and ovaries removed because of life-threatening hemorrhaging after a car accident. As a result her body is deprived of estrogen, which increases her risk for osteoporosis. She also develops insomnia, emotional instability, and a range of physical problems resulting from the hormone loss. These short-term problems are resolved with a prescription for estrogen, and her long-term risk for osteoporosisis reduced.

She is replacing a natural hormone produced by the body with a natural hormone produced by the body. Does it matter if she thinks she's on a drug rather than viewing the medication as the hormone transplant it actually is? Absolutely.

After all, she can never have her own children, she has an ugly scar on her tummy at the age of 20, and she struggles with nightmares about the accident. If she believes she's being further penalized with a drug that may be risky, toxic, or unnatural, she is more likely to flatly refuse the treatment.

On the other hand, if she thinks of it as the natural replacement of estrogen, she is more likely to want to actively participate in the decision- making process, to learn about and weigh all the risks and benefits. Then, her decision will be based on a real, informed understanding instead of an emotional misperception.

From one point of view, estrogen pills are seen as a medicinal punishment for losing her reproductive organs. In another context, they represent the action of a powerful person "taking back" what was stolen prematurely from her life. When she uses the medication, she feels more like her old self; the integrity of her bones and her mood is maintained, as is her normal, youthful appearance. She also has a more natural, comfortable sexual response. But, she is still using a substance to deliberately alter the way she feels or how her body functions. She's on a drug.

What other deliberate actions do we undertake to alter our own chemistry and create a desired physiologic effect? Almost everything.

Thanks to modern laboratory tests and imaging technologies such as Positron Emission Tomography (PET) and Magnetic Resonance Imaging (MRI), we now know that hundreds of *normal* activities have the same effects on our bodies and brains as medications or recreational drugs.

We know alcohol, coffee, and tobacco alter our physiology. That first cup of coffee is the high point of my day, and I wouldn't give it up willingly without a very good reason.

Modern scanners can now show the effect of caffeine from our coffee, soda, or no-doze pills; we actually "see" the effect of this drug on our brains and bodies as noradrenaline and dopamine levels rise. They can show the drug effect when a hungry person eats bread as the neurons that release serotonin become more active. Serotonin is a neurotransmitter that affects our moods. When released by specific brain cells, the subjective feeling of the person scanned is one of contentment, a direct response to eating carbohydrates. Bread, cake, and cookies *really are* comfort foods, things we turn to for a reward or to help us cope during a stressful time.

Does this mean we are drugging our kids with a cupcake? You bet. But not in any criminal way. *Any* food can be considered a drug, because when we eat, our body's chemistry is altered. When we are hungry, we have higher levels of circulating adrenaline, making us energetic and more than a little fierce. Low blood sugar releases hormones to mobilize stored energy and prompt us to eat; the hunter is uncaged. As soon as we get some food in us, the signals are reversed, calming the "warrior status" of our bodies and minds.

Have you ever noticed irritable customers waiting for a table at a restaurant and how they quickly begin to love life after the food and drink are served? So in a broad sense, it could be argued that everything we ingest is a drug. But it doesn't stop there.

Some chemicals we inhale have profound drug effects. Not just negative things like pollens and gas fumes, but pleasant things as well. Stopping to smell roses stimulates the sensation of pleasure and causes us to come back for more the next time we encounter the flower. Is this drug-seeking behavior? Sure, a harmless one.

Some of the most powerful inhaled drugs aren't even noticed with our conscious minds. Pheromones, for instance, are naturally-occurring molecules secreted by humans that have a drug-like effect on other humans. Many of the details of pheromones and their effects are still a mystery; however, we know they play a role in the physical attraction between men and women.

A newborn baby, cuddled close to your neck and face, provides a powerful, indefinable scent that can give you a giddy high. Our bodies produce inhalant drugs that bond us to each other.

A faint aroma once caught my attention when I was walking in the small resort town of Sedona, Arizona. I couldn't identify it, but I was compelled to follow it. Down the block, I recognized some elements of the smell and thought it might be the enticing scent of fresh-brewed coffee. Then I was at the door of the source—a chocolate shop. A vat of hot, dark fudge was being poured into a mold. The windows were wide open, a fan blowing the shop's air out into the streets. No accident, I'm sure.

I lost my intense interest in the scent once I found its source, but I had been drawn to it involuntarily. Part of the craving for chocolate may very well be that it mimics nearly irresistible human sexual pheromones.

It goes further. Our brains react to many non-chemical signals in the same way we respond to pills, foods, drinks, smokes, and smells. Sunlight is a powerful drug. First, it's an essential source for vitamin D production. It's also among the better antidepressants in the world. Who hasn't felt that sudden sense of well-being when the clouds lift to reveal brilliant blue skies? Who hasn't experienced a slump in mood on cloudy days? George Harrison's, "Here comes the Sun," is a song most of us "get."

While we're on the subject of songs, what about music itself? When I don't get my daily "fix" of music, I get grumpy. My spirits lift immediately when I hear a song I like and drop if the next song is one I don't.

We've talked about the drug effects of smell, taste, sight, and sound. What other senses affect our brain-chemistry? Certainly touch counts. At our house, back scratches and head massages are highly valued currencies of exchange.

Psychiatrists know sex is a powerful drug, normally a healthy one, but for some people, addictive. A combination of senses as well as social feedback can also act like a drug. Consider the "thrill seeker." People labeled as "attention deficit disordered" often seek high-speed racing or other extreme sensations as a form of self-medication. There are stage performers who can't get enough applause. What about the gambler, whose occasional big wins are addictive enough to lead him back to the gaming tables again and again until he's lost everything? Fishing remains an enigma to many hard-working wives, but can be a reward unrivaled for many hard-working husbands. And we guys don't all "get" shopping, but we can sense its power.

Some of these hidden drugs don't produce pleasure but are just as strong. The sound of one's baby crying can produce a surge of feelings: fear, concern, doubt, and yes, frustration. It can also start the flow of a mother's breast milk.

The sight of a creepy insect or slithering snake can cause instant, involuntary fear and revulsion. Too many males or females together in competing circumstances can exaggerate grievances, fire up tempers, or just synchronize menstrual cycles.

My list of "hidden drugs" is always growing. Here are a few:

Sunshine • Music • Coffee • The scent of a baby • Chocolate • Ocean Waves • Petting a Puppy • Sex • Ice Cream • Shopping • Television • Landing a Fish • Skydiving • Applause • "Miller Time" • Runner's "High" • Dancing • Sculpting, and, as you've probably guessed, Writing.

More destructive hidden drugs might include:

Tobacco use • Feeling Power or Dominance through Rape or Beating • Gambling • Thrilling to the Danger of Burglary, Robbery or even Murder • Heroin • Child Molestation • Compulsive Plastic Surgery.

What would you put on your list?

From one point of view, it is reasonable to consider most things we choose to do as having some drug-like effect. We act, deliberately or unconsciously, to create brain responses such as pleasure or to achieve a goal. We also act, deliberately or subconsciously, to avoid pain, sadness, anxiety, and other unpleasant feelings. To say "I don't ever use drugs," from my point of view, would be like saying "I'm dead."

Why is chocolate cake more acceptable than Prozac? Why is an addiction to coffee okay, but an addiction to heroin criminal? What makes a drug healthy or dangerous? If your answers are based on half-truths, myths, or a broad, biased definition, you're effectively uninformed. And that means unnecessary risk to your health and well-being.

"In the future, maybe nicotine will become illegal, probably about the same time that medical marijuana is sold by prescription at your corner pharmacy."

Chapter 5

Good Drug – Bad Drug

Addiction.

My patients, like many of you, are fearful of becoming dependent on a drug. They fear they won't be able to give it up, that it could destroy their lives. The devastation of drug addiction is real, of course, but its portrayal in films, TV, literature, and the daily news has burned a fear of it into our collective psyche.

When I was in high school, cocaine was reported in the news as a recreational drug with very few problems for users. Before that, Valium—mother's little helper. Before that, thalidomide—the safest sleeping pill of its day and the origin of countless birth defects. The knowledge of such fiascos can convince otherwise logical and concerned patients to avoid safe medications that could save or significantly prolong their lives.

So, what makes a drug bad? Is it the horrors of withdrawal, of physical dependency? There can be worse things. I prescribe essential, life-saving heart medications upon which the body becomes so dependent, it becomes dangerous to stop the drugs abruptly. However, for the patients on these drugs, the much bigger danger is in *not* starting them in the first place.

You will probably tell me with great conviction that heroin and cocaine are bad drugs. I would agree—in most cases. Using them for recreation is a deadly game; once you're hooked, giving them up is physical, emotional, and mental torture, remaining a struggle for the rest your life.

Imagine being totally exhausted but unable to rest or sleep. Or being completely wound up and agitated but utterly unable to actually *do* anything except feel anxious, nauseated, and wretched. Withdrawal is awful.

Yet, there are few topical anesthetics better than cocaine for numbing the inside of the nose during nasal surgery. Not only does it alleviate pain, it helps control bleeding as well. Heroin itself is not used in medicine, but its sister drugs are the mainstay of pain control.

Fortunately, public perception of cigarettes has finally evolved from cool and seductive to nasty. They're bad for the health of both smokers and second-hand smokers, and they're addictive. On the other hand, you don't see too many road raging maniacs shooting up the freeway while enjoying a cigarette. Smokers have long used tobacco pacifiers to manage through traffic jams, intense or chronic stress, and other potentially explosive situations.

Am I suggesting you start smoking? Of course not. What we're doing here is re-thinking the assumptions that any drug is all good or all bad.

So, of course, we come to alcohol - merciless killer and home wrecker or harmless social lubricant? I guess your answer depends on the decade from which you're answering the question. During prohibition, alcohol was considered a grave and criminal evil. Today, children in France start having wine with dinner at a very young age and, apparently, are at lower risk for alcohol abuse. We read about research showing people who have three glasses of red wine per week living longer with fewer heart attacks.

In the future, nicotine may become illegal, probably about the same time that medical marijuana is sold by prescription at your corner pharmacy.

What are the societal differences between marijuana and alcohol? One major distinction is that marijuana is illegal and alcohol is not. Yet from a drug standpoint, *both* are habit-forming for some people; both can cause physical, medical, and social problems. Either one would be a bad idea before getting on the freeway at rush hour.

So, why might one drug be accepted as legal and another not? For one thing, *anyone* can brew alcohol in their home, as the failed experiment of prohibition demonstrated so well. Besides, it has been part of civilizations for millennia. Wine making, the brewing of beer, and the distillation of spirits are regarded as high art forms. Jesus himself made wine in the Bible story.

Marijuana is easy to grow and use. It has legitimate medicinal purposes for many forms of human suffering and weighs in as a *mildly illegal* drug. Heroin is very addictive. So is cocaine with its associated cardiac risks. Both take work and knowledge to purify and prepare. Both are *very illegal*.

Yet heroin, while terribly addictive, is not itself especially toxic. Heroin deaths are usually related to impure drugs of unknown strength and to contaminated needles. Its victims are primarily people living in poverty, which comes with its own inherent health risks. Pure heroin, in controlled daily doses, is actually safer that cigarettes.

Because of the huge legal risk, drugs like heroin are expensive, profitable, and often linked to crime; while, to the best of my knowledge, nobody ever robbed a convenience store or killed a stranger for enough cash to "score" a pack of cigarettes. But, nicotine cravings and the price of dope aside, more *innocent* people have been killed by drunk drivers and second-hand smoke than from stoned drivers and junkies.

While alcohol and tobacco have taken a greater toll than all the others combined, all of these—alcohol, tobacco, marijuana, heroin, and cocaine—are considered recreational drugs, because they alter the body's state of consciousness for pleasure. The illegality or acceptability of a recreational drug, then, is more a product of history, politics, availability, and marketing than of the hedonistic reasons for its use.

No question, getting involved with mind-altering substances is grabbing a tiger by the tail. It doesn't make a difference whether it is sold in the back alleys of the inner city, at the liquor store, or by your friendly pharmacist with a doctor's note and FDA approval. A potentially habit-forming drug can be psychologically dangerous to one person and be neutral or beneficial for another. They are what they are. And whether we outlaw them, and so create a booming black market, or legalize them and collect taxes from their use, they will always be here. It's our responsibility to personally avoid drugs that endanger our well-being and that of others. It's also our responsibility to know when a potentially addictive drug can be used safely and to our benefit.

Remember those *natural* remedies - herbs and supplements? Chemically, there is no difference between prescription drugs from the drugstore and non-prescription products from the health food store used for medicinal purposes. Both are drugs. The primary difference is that prescription drugs almost always have two things herbs and "food supplements" do not: a substantial body of expensive research to determine their safety and effectiveness, and a patent protecting the rights of those who developed and funded that substantial body of research.

Herbs are simply non-patented, non-prescription drugs, often with little or no research about their effects on the human body. These drugs hide behind the more lenient laws governing food supplements. Not only is there nothing intrinsically safer about herb capsules in a bottle, there are actually fewer safeguards for consumers.

When a prescription drug arrives on the market, it means that about a decade or so earlier a patent was filed on a biological substance (naturally occurring or synthetic), or on a processing technology for making the compound usable for treatment. Then, hundreds of millions of dollars are spent testing and retesting for safety, side-effects, therapeutic uses, routes of delivery (pills, injections, creams, etc.), interactions with other medications, and much more.

Then, if the research supports the drug's benefits and quantifies its safety to be acceptable, the FDA scrutinizes the quality and documentation of each clinical result. That can take several more years.

After this lengthy and rigorous process, clinicians know a lot about the drug, including who should take it and who should not, how much and for how long, and what to expect from treatment.

The company that invests hundreds of millions in research to get a patented product from laboratory to patient has to recoup its investment. The company that sells an unpatented herb does not, and therefore will not spend big money on researching their product's safety and benefits. Even if they wanted to, without exclusive sales rights, such spending would be financial suicide. I wish our government would spend a bit of *its* research funds to scientifically evaluate the major herbal "remedies." Fewer people would pay the price of using ineffective remedies for serious illnesses, and truly effective supplements could proudly boast their own merits.

Until then, herbal remedies remain classified as "food supplements." You won't see specific, binding medicinal claims on most herbal medicine bottles because, by law, specific health effects cannot be claimed for food supplements without solid research evidence.

Yet I've never met anyone who uses St. John's Wort because it tastes good on his tofu. It's used as a drug, based on assertions that it acts as a mild antidepressant. It may or may not live up to the claim. The point is that insufficient clinical evidence exists to prove it is safe and effective and, if it is, in what doses and for which patients.

The medicinal claims that drive supplement consumption come indirectly, from word-of-mouth or published articles by supposedly non-affiliated advocates. Yet some herbs and vitamins can be as potent as any prescription drug both in medical value and in side-effects. Large amounts of Vitamin A can destroy your liver, and an allergic reaction to bee pollen (yeah, the health food store stuff) can be deadly. On the other hand, niacin in high doses is clearly a cardiac life-saver for some patients.

Even when prescription medications are clinically shown to be safe and effective, the manufacturer must monitor for "adverse events" in thousands of patients, usually over a period of years. Even if bad experiences have nothing to do with the medication, prescriptions drug makers must collect data on all *possible* side-effects.

Have you ever noticed that what we focus on becomes bigger in our lives? The energy we focus on these side-effects, both real and potential, can draw our attention mainly to the risks, not the benefits, of using a medication, thereby leading to the unfounded perception that it's more dangerous to use a prescription drug than an herbal medicine, a substance that has not been rigorously tested for safety.

If 20 million Americans take Echinacea and 1,000 of them (about .005 percent) develop a heart or lung disease, who would know about it? Would anyone ever notice or be able to make a connection between the herb and the disease?

But a pickup even more rare led to the 1997 withdrawal from the market of the weight loss medications Redux and fenfluramine—the latter was half of the infamous Phen-Fen combination.

Today, almost a decade later, debate continues as to how much these drugs contributed to the lung and heart diseases they were blamed for and how much was caused by obesity itself. I think the preponderance of evidence points to yes, the drugs caused heart and/or lung damage in some patients. If so, this means we were able to pick a needle out of a haystack—only 24 initial cases out of 19 million prescriptions—because of the monitoring associated with the use of prescription medications.

One fact the media doesn't go out of their way to share is that for every fenfluramine or Vioxx that gets pulled from the market, there are thousands of prescription medications that have withstood, for decades, the searing scrutiny of the safety watchdogs.

What about health food supplements? Have any turned out to be dangerous? Ah, the wonders of Ephedra. For decades, emergency room doctors across America watched people die from this "all natural" speed before it was banned by the FDA in 2003. We're not talking about .005 percent here.

The toxicity was so compelling, there was no question within the medical community that people could and would kill themselves with this drug. Yet a quick search of the web today reveals many websites defending Ephedra as a safe and (no surprise) *all natural* energy or weight loss "supplement." These non-medical, non-scientific and, in my mind unethical commercial sites are promoting lifting the ban on a natural killer.

Phen-Fen was yanked off the market within a few weeks of making headlines, while it took decades to ban a deadly herb. Phen-Fen vanished with virtually no discussion of the lost benefits to millions of overweight people. If I had to choose one, I'd take Phen-Fen over Ephedra in *my* diet any day.

But Phen-Fen was a story made in TV-ratings heaven. It captured audiences with over-the-top, sensationalized news. Americans are obsessed with both weight loss and the danger of drugs, and 20 million Americans were taking fenfluramine or its cousin Redux.

Now add to this our often harsh and biased attitudes toward the obese. I saw no fair or balanced reporting on the benefits of Phen-Fen. Even though an overweight person may suffer from relentless back, hip, knee, and foot pain, or endure diabetic complications like kidney failure, leg amputation, and blindness, relying on pills instead of willpower to help avoid these things is often judged as going too far.

Many in our society relish corporate scandals and misfortune, especially those of pharmaceutical companies. News producers and editors play to this audience segment, because it's a large one and because it's so much easier to just report one side of a story.

Interestingly, there's no public outrage about companies profiting from unproven weight loss meals, drinks, super foods, natural supplements, fat-burning equipment, miracle-diets, or exclusive "fat farms."

It's a multi-billion dollar industry selling to our society's genuine problem with unhealthy weight gain. Companies that prey on this market, without needing to prove product safety or efficacy, dread the potential of an effective pharmaceutical solution.

Fenfluramine and Redux were removed from the market voluntarily by their manufacturers. Phentermine, the drug paired with fenfluramine, was never suspected of the same problems and is still available. The companies knew that regardless of the facts, bad press and the panic that resulted would make it extremely difficult to get a fair hearing in any personal or class-action lawsuit.

More recently, "breaking news" stories fueled panic among those taking the anti-inflammatory drugs, Vioxx or Bextra, for arthritis pain.

The manufacturers of these drugs also took their products off the market voluntarily. As with the diet pills, there is credible information suggesting that these medications increase risk for heart attack or stroke in some patients. *Some* patients. And physicians have the knowledge and tools to identify patients who should not take Vioxx or Bextra.

Ben and Jerry's and Häagen-Dazs products are still on the market, available to people of all ages, even though they increase risk for obesity and heart disease. And they don't even alleviate the pain of arthritis!

Here's an interesting fact about Vioxx and Bextra that was seldom addressed in the media frenzy: While on the market, these medications were usually prescribed as substitutes for over-the-counter arthritis medications that kill thousands of people every year by causing bleeding stomach ulcers.

Vioxx and Bextra are well known to be less toxic to the stomach lining and have a better net life-saving track record compared to their over-the-counter counterparts. Yet no one is demanding that ibuprofen, aspirin, and naproxen be pulled from the market despite their serious side-effects on the gastrointestinal system.

Let me be clear. I don't want those products taken off the shelves. And I'd be devastated if they banned ice cream. My message is that you need to look beyond the headlines, seek a broader and more informed perspective on issues that have a role in your health decisions. Very few health issues are so simple they can be explained in sound bites. It takes time and effort, but it *is* your life and well-being we're talking about.

My patients, like many others, lost the benefits of Vioxx and Bextra overnight, and many have no equivalent treatment for their arthritis pain. Removal of Vioxx and Bextra means they will be more limited in physical activity which diminishes their conditioning and balance. Their risk for a disabling fall increases, and their cardiovascular risk may be greater, as a result of inactivity, than it would be from taking either of the drugs.

Many patients will also turn to older medications that cause more stomach bleeding. The inability for physicians to discriminately prescribe Vioxx and Bextra has an overall negative impact on the health and well-being of patients with arthritis

It is a frustrating situation when medications that greatly reduce suffering are taken away as a result of public fear, politics, and the potential for litigation. In many cases, physicians can successfully mitigate the drug's small risk with close management of coexisting cardiac risk factors —something they should be doing anyway. Would I still be prescribing Vioxx for my patients if it were still available? You Bet.

So where are we in the vast gray area between all good and all bad in the world of "official," recreational and "food supplement" drugs?

▶ **The fact that alcohol is legal and socially acceptable doesn't make it all good. The belief that marijuana is all bad, all the time, for all people, limits its accessibility for people who would greatly benefit from its role in cancer treatment and alleviating severe, chronic pain.**

▶ **All drugs have biological effects, sometimes useful, sometimes destructive, often both, but their value and risk should be based on careful research—never solely on the news of the day.**

▶ **Refusing a prescription drug because it didn't sprout in your garden is not good for your health and may reduce your time on earth.**

▶ **If you choose to use herbal products, mega-vitamins, or other supplements, do so with your eyes open. Understand that most of their direct or indirect claims of benefit have not been proven and that reliable information about their safety or recommended dosage does not exist. That doesn't mean they don't have value or aren't safe. It means we don't know.**

Living *is* a risk. Drugs, prescription, herbal, or recreational, can kill people. So can driving. So can dessert. Fear and overreacting does not lower that risk, but ignorance *does* increase it.

I'm not championing all conventional medications, and I'm not condemning all alternative healthcare—in practice, I refer to acupuncturists, prescribe a variety of supplements, and in general promote a team approach to wellness—but I *am* asking you to be an informed healthcare consumer and actively participate in decisions about the content and scope of that care. I believe the best kind of "alternative medicine" is *Think-For-Yourself-Medicine* based on informed, reasoned consideration of the best available knowledge.

Are you calmly weighing all available information on a subject, taking into account any important facts you *do not yet know*, recognizing when you are forming opinions based on illogical beliefs, fears or emotions?

Think-For-Yourself-Medicine also means ignoring skewed advertising messages and identifying the hype and one-sided reporting we so often find in our sensationalized news reports. The first step in doing so will be to *consider the source* of our information. Most of us get our ideas about what's healthy, safe, toxic, or fattening from the nightly news media, popular magazines, and from consumer advertising. The key is to respond with skepticism, looking behind the scenes for what you are really being "sold"—and for who's doing the selling.

BAD DATA

*"One day you hear coffee can add years to your life;
the next day it's reported to cause prostate cancer.
Is it possible that it does both?"*

Chapter 6

Consider the Source

"HEY DOC, I JUST HEARD… EGGS ARE KILLING PEOPLE!
VIOXX IS KILLING PEOPLE. EVERYONE'S LOSING WEIGHT
ON THAT ALL-PROTEIN DIET. EVERYONE'S DYING FROM
THAT ALL-PROTEIN DIET! EXERCISE INCREASES MY CHANCE
OF A HEART ATTACK. BUT LACK OF EXERCISE INCREASES
MY CHANCE OF ALZHEIMER DISEASE. ALCOHOL KILLS BRAIN
CELLS. BUT A GLASS OF WINE EVERY DAY WILL HELP ME
LIVE LONGER—BUT WITHOUT A BRAIN? MY ANTI-
DEPRESSANT CAUSED A WOMAN TO SHOOT HER HUSBAND
ON THEIR 40TH ANNIVERSARY!"

Some days I know how the White House press team must feel when performing their frantic damage control. My phone starts to ring within minutes of a breaking news story about a medical threat that will kill us or a new breakthrough that will grant eternal life.

Sometimes patients want to reserve their dose of whichever vaccine is suddenly in short supply or an antibiotic prescription for the impending anthrax attack. Most of the time, however, they want to know if they should flush away their prescription medication based on the latest news horror story. I'm glad for those calls, because often the worst thing patients could do is toss their medication without telling me.

We know what drives broadcast news. Ratings. We know what drives print media. Advertising sales. Because of these two driving forces, the media seldom provide news we can actually use. This has serious implications for anyone who considers the news media a reliable source for health information.

Many people now rely almost solely on television to know what's going on in the world. The most effective way to hang onto this huge audience is to give them sensationalized teasers. **Is Your Drinking Water Safe? Kansas Boy Dies After taking Ritalin!** *Are We Just Days Away From Armageddon?*

By the very nature of broadcast news, viewers get only a fleeting glimpse of an issue, 30 seconds—maybe a whole minute, that merely skims the surface of the facts, missing some altogether. Producers, facing fierce competition for viewers, are compelled to grab attention quickly and hold onto it for dear life. Thus, sensationalized headlines and the stories that follow are barely appetizers with just a tad of substance to justify the packaging. Network and cable news cannot afford the whole meal; they know spending adequate time on a subject will have their antsy viewers reaching for the remote.

We cannot get the whole story if our only source for current information is the Nightly News or Good Morning, America. Credible newspapers and the Internet have the luxury of being less hurried, so they *could* offer more details, greater depth, and the opportunity to consider both sides of an issue—only a benefit if one takes the time to read the whole story, of course. And even then, important facts are often missing, distorted, or over-simplified while drama is splashed across the front page to hook us. The newspaper industry, after all, coined the expression, "If it bleeds, it leads."

There is also no way to get balanced news from a publication or website with its own agenda or political or financial bias. If your only source for news is the Polygamist Daily or KKK Weekly, you will not be wholly informed.

I doubt I'm telling you anything you don't already know. But there's an interesting twist here when it comes to health issues. When you watch a politician being interviewed about an issue like illegal immigration or his opponent's tax plan, you apply your innate skepticism. You filter his opinion through your brain's *Yeah, Right* filter. Even if you agree with him, you know he has an agenda.

But what happens when a newscaster announces breathlessly that a child in Kansas dies seconds after taking his first dose of Ritalin? Many people forget to use their filters. Because the subject is *health*, not politics, they're inclined to accept the information as fact – the whole truth and nothing but.

In this case, parents whose children are being treated for ADHD are immediately alarmed. On the screen, a glimpse of grieving parents, an old clip of Tom Cruise, and a heart-wrenching photo of the little boy playing soccer. The attorney for the devastated parents announces a lawsuit against the manufacturer. By the time a medical expert explains there is no evidence of any relationship between the Ritalin and the boy's fatal asthma attack, people have already formed their opinion.

One day you hear coffee can add years to your life; the next day it's reported to cause prostate cancer. We get contradictions and inconsistencies every day from myriad sources. Information is skewed to emphasize only the part of the story or promotion most likely to command our attention. Is it possible that coffee causes prostate cancer AND may add years to your life? Sure. I don't believe coffee has been proven to do either one, but stories of this kind can provide accurate facts and still leave us effectively uninformed, unable to decide whether to go with the latte or the bottled water.

Please, activate your skepticism every time the news focuses on health issues. When you hear your prescribed drug is being scrutinized for whatever reason, call your doctor *before* you stop taking the medication. Every day, someone suffers serious consequences by stopping or self-adjusting a prescribed treatment.

> *"Thousands already use this widely prescribed medication which is a billion-dollar boon for WILEY LABORATORIES, the pharmaceutical giant that sells it. But W-IRD has the exclusive on its deadly impact for thousands of people. Are you one of them? Join us at 11:00 for all the details."*
> W-IRD Nightly News with Willy Hype

Fear-based headlines, strategically placed within primetime viewing, coerce us to stay tuned. I'm sure we've all hung in there, compelled to watch some story that caught our attention, only to come away feeling the actual report was no more informative than the commercial teaser that grabbed our attention.

When we are *compelled* to do something, we are not in control. For example, the weeks following the 9/11 nightmare saw millions of stressed out viewers glued to their sets, literally unable to turn them off. Replayed scenes of death, horror, and grief scorched their emotional and physical health. By two weeks after the attack, half a dozen patients came to me with anxiety, insomnia, and depression, and every one of them still had their TV sets spewing trauma into their lives.

As soon as they agreed to unplug their sets, they began to heal. We each must deal with our own portion of life's grief and pain, but we were not built to *also* feel the suffering of millions of other people while being excluded from feeling their joys. This is why I no longer get my news from TV producers who have pre-digested it for their viewers.

Fear is also held in high esteem by advertisers. Plato taught that pain and pleasure are the two primary human motivators; masters in marketing know that the best attention-grabbing hooks embody elements of one or both. In the hands of a pro, they can help sell just about anything to anyone. On that basis, my top three picks for the best "marketing emotions" are these: GREED, LUST and FEAR.

Do you sense any negative emotion when you read these words? I know I do. In a famous scene from the movie "Wall Street," Michael Douglas, as Gordon Gekko, states he lives by the creed that "Greed is Great." Yet many of us were raised to believe that greed is shameful, a source of evil. And Lust? A culture that demands its members to feel guilt from basic, natural urges leaves those members oppressed and vulnerable to their own longings.

Regardless of how we feel about Greed and Lust, they get our attention. And why shouldn't they? They're part of us. Mother Nature made sure of that. Greed draws us to the things we need to keep a roof over our head, food on the table, and even to be successful enough to find a mate—now we're back to Lust. These natural human traits have long played their parts in civilization, but now their cultivation by "spin doctors" is in overdrive.

Our entire society has been shaped by mass manufacturing, mass merchandising, and mass media to make us always want more than we have. Fueling greed is what has made our country the richest in the world. And, like it or not, sex permeates every aspect of our being. The power of greed and lust are beautifully reflected in the booming industry that sells them to us day in and day out—advertising.

And let's not forget Fear, perhaps the most prevalent, visceral American emotion of the 21st century. On September 11, our baby boomer assumptions about living in a nation safe from attack were annihilated along with the victims in the Twin Towers and all four doomed airliners. Now, the realization that our Land of the Free is vulnerable to unspeakable acts joins the list of everyday fears like growing old, suffering, dying, abandonment, poverty, and public speaking.

Our entertainment, personal priorities, and political discussions reflect this. Look at the content of movies, television, books, and even our Internet SPAM. Reality shows like Fear Factor are light and airy compared to the disturbing, brutal violence portrayed in the forensic dramas that fill prime time.

Fear has always been a major catalyst of sales, but today's marketplace may go down as the most paranoia-driven economy since atomic fallout shelters were popular sellers.

Right now I hope you're thinking: *Hey, wait a minute! This guy hooked me into reading this book because he knows I'm afraid of dying! And I guess he also knows I don't want to die of stupidity!* True. Most likely, you picked up this book because you were intrigued by the title (or else you're a dutiful member of my family.)

The use of Greed, Lust or Fear to catch somebody's attention isn't good or bad, nor is it the exclusive domain of sleazy advertising. It's how we function. We offer a raise to keep a good employee, we dress up and flirt to attract a mate, and we hope our kids are terrified of getting into a car with a stranger.

In advertising, Fear is also employed because it can be integral to more positive emotions. Headlines promising greater beauty actually play on our fear of rejection, those promising wealth, on our fear of poverty, and the chance for a longer life (yes, like this book) play on our fear of death.

▶ **LOSE FIVE DRESS SIZES BY BIKINI SEASON!**

▶ **ARTHRITIS ACHES AND PAINS WILL DISAPPEAR WHEN YOU TAKE THIS NEW, ALL-NATURAL WONDER DRUG!**

▶ **THE CANCER CURE YOUR DOCTOR WON'T TELL YOU ABOUT!**

If only I had a dollar for every cure I was supposed to be keeping a secret. The next time you notice a health claim on a product label ask yourself, "What have they left out?"

Truth-in-advertising laws prevent outright lying, but nobody's forced to tell the whole truth. I once encountered an orange juice carton which proudly displayed: "Contains Vitamin C!" In smaller letters it read: *"Vitamin C may lower your risk of cancer"*.

There actually are some statistical associations between the use of vitamins in general and life span. The group of all people who take vitamins is known to live longer, but that's because they're health-conscious people in the first place. Those who can afford to drop a lot of cash at health food stores tend not to be smokers, prostitutes, or heroin addicts and live well above the poverty line. They represent a generally healthier subset of the American population. Associations of this type mean nothing except, perhaps, increased sales.

A cause and effect relationship between Vitamin C and a reduced chance of cancer could only be demonstrated by enrolling thousands of people into a study and following them for many years. Half would receive high doses of vitamin C and half would receive a placebo instead. The two groups would need to be similar in all other respects: age distribution, gender mix, percentage of smokers, average weight, etc. The study would be "double-blind," meaning that no one, not the test subjects nor the researchers, would know who got what. The incidence of cancer would be measured in the whole group, and a computer would sort it all out at the end.

It's a lot of work and a lot of money. It's been done on a small scale several times. The verdict: no direct connection between vitamin C consumption and a longer life or fewer cancers has ever been demonstrated.

Now, let's get back to our delicious orange juice. Time to check your reality filters. What's left off the label is the fact that *no proof* of cancer prevention actually exists. Remember, the carton said it "*may*" lower your risk. Which means it may not.

But let's say Vitamin C *was* proven to lower risk for cancer. Is that enough to sell you on the orange juice? Wouldn't you want to know if your risk of cancer will be lowered by 90 percent or one-tenth of one percent? How much orange juice would you need to reach that percentage? A glass? A gallon? If you're diabetic, drinking a gallon of o.j. might just put you into a coma, in which case the risk of cancer is not your biggest problem.

Which cancers are we talking about? If it's only prostate cancer, the claim doesn't apply to about half the human race. And could we get an even better effect from other foods or from a different brand of orange juice?

What about the ever-popular "low-fat" and "no-cholesterol" claims plastered on products? Great big letters. Teeny tiny meaning. Many people remain unaware that without fat and cholesterol we would die, or that our blood cholesterol level itself is largely irrelevant to our heart disease risk. But we do know there exists *some* relationship between fats, cholesterol, and death. Advertisers know it all too well, and *they* know that *you* know.

They know there is a substantial market for Sadie's delicious, non-fat coffee cake. Their ad campaign doesn't mention all the sugar and salt in Sadie's recipe. Same with no-cholesterol products that are loaded with saturated fats which are *not* good for you

A jar of peanut butter or tub of margarine is promoted as "cholesterol-free." Unless you have a degree in biology, you might not know that all brands of peanut butter and margarine are cholesterol-free. Consumers may think that since butter has cholesterol and margarine doesn't, that margarine must be a healthier. No research even remotely supports that assumption.

Our minds have never been entirely our own. We manipulate each other. We always have. That's what it means to be social creatures. Today the science that goes into influencing human behavior is as sophisticated as the technological hardware that disseminates it. Subliminal coercion works well. Really well.

There have always been good natural salesmen on the planet, but the past century has seen the systematic study and implementation of techniques that not only affect our buying and voting behavior but that have transformed our entire culture to one based primarily on consumption.

Author, Douglas Rushkoff, provides an unnerving look behind the scenes of human manipulation in his book, *Coercion: Why We Listen To What "They" Say.*

> *"Coercion seeks to stymie our rational processes in order to make us act against—or, at least, without—our better judgment. Once immersed in a coercive system, we act without conscious control. We act automatically, from a place that has little to do with reason."* [2]

He traces modern sales and media techniques from the mom and pop general store, where needed merchandise was all that brought customers to spend their hard-earned money, through the creation of shopping malls, designed to disorient the consumer to yield greater sales, on up to the overpowering experience of a visit to the Flagship Nike Store in New York City, a destination theme park in itself. What do car salesmen and CIA interrogators have in common? In fact, how is *my* pointing out to you the manipulations we all face, in and of itself, a form of manipulation? Troubling stuff.

The more aware you are of being coerced, the smarter choices you will make about what is truly healthy and what isn't, because you'll ignore more hype and demand more facts.

This is not to say that *all* the information that comes to us through the media or advertising is deceptive or manipulative. My point is that advertising claims should never form the basis for any health decision.

What would happen if the world of media and advertising suddenly found itself controlled by some dreadful "fact police"? Imagine, broadcasters too frightened to express any opinion or emotion as they reported pure, dry data. If anyone bothered to watch, would they better understand the truth behind the facts? Maybe not. Recognizing the gimmicks of ratings and advertising, and using our "skeptic filters" are important skills. But that only addresses half the problem.

When it comes to Bad Data, *we* are the other half of the problem. Confusion and misinformation also surface in everyday human interactions. With the best intention, people often get facts *partly* wrong when they pass on to another person something they heard or read. When your friend, relative, co-worker, or hair stylist updates you on the latest health news, keep in mind that the likelihood of inaccuracy and missing facts is huge. The truth may have started with a solid scientific study, made it into a respected medical journal and then been condensed by the media. Your "source" condenses it even more based on what they remember, what they think about it, and how it fits into their reality. In other words, don't believe every thing you hear, even from sources whose motives you trust.

Progress in medicine, especially in the areas of wellness and prevention, comes to us in the form of *statistical* data. And most of us don't really "do" statistics. My former school teacher, a very smart lady, once taught our class if "heads" had come up five times in a row on a coin toss, that it would make more sense to bet on "tails" for the next flip.

It doesn't. But instinctively the concept *feels* right. After all, a coin can't come up heads forever, can it? When human instinct colors our interpretation of scientific information, mistakes happen. Add to this our cultural distrust of science, and it's no wonder that millions turn their backs on information and technology that could add years to their lives. It's a shame, since science and technology really aren't the bad guys when it comes to preventing and curing disease.

*"So which doctor is right? The one who's quick to prescribe
a drug and doesn't seem to care about killing your liver?
Or the other, who has faith in you to 'get healthy'
and is willing to let you die trying?"*

Chapter 7

High Tech – High Stakes

Make no mistake, Vioxx *did* kill some people. Lipitor still does. Familiar drugs, household names, can occasionally take a living, breathing man or woman and make them dead. So why would I frequently prescribe Lipitor and wish Vioxx was still available? Because, from a scientific point of view, these choices make the most sense for specific patients. Because the net effect of both these drugs is to *save* lives.

Science and technology are powerful forces in our lives—often beneficial, sometimes hazardous. The trick is in understanding how to use them for the most benefit with the least possible risk.

It's easy to think all technology has run amok. Fluorocarbons punched a hole in our ozone, and global warming threatens to melt Antarctica. We've doubled the carbon dioxide in our air by burning fossil fuels, the lynch pin of a global civilization. Species continue to disappear from the planet. Nuclear waste piles up with nowhere to go. We may even unleash nuclear power to destroy civilization some day. No question, some of the products of science and technology are as dreadful as anything Mother Nature ever created.

The combined global impact of the industrial age, plus six billion people, amounts to a clumsy science experiment on our only home. The changes we've imposed on Earth cannot be undone. We'll have to live with the consequences. No second chances.

Modern medicine, built on the foundation of science and technology, must share this legacy of fear and mismanagement. It has a dark side. But there is also a clear difference between the applied technology that gives us global warming and that which gives us video surgery,

MRI scanners, and prescription drugs. In the world of medical research we *do* get second chances. We repeat experiments over and over, adjusting each time based on the results until we get it as close to "right" as possible.

In the development of a new drug, initial testing is done in laboratories, first on cells, then on animals. (I'm not taking sides on the animal rights controversy, these are just the facts.) Once there is evidence of safety and medical value, the drug is tested in a small group of closely-monitored human volunteers, then in a slightly larger group to confirm safety and evaluate its effectiveness. Then, larger clinical studies are conducted at major research centers. This process may take well over a decade. Along with re-confirming safety and effectiveness in larger populations, medical investigators focus on appropriate dosages, methods of administrating the drug, side-effects, and interactions with other medications. Modern medicines are tested more extensively than most foods we eat every day.

Mary hates the idea of taking a prescription drug. Reluctantly, she agrees to start one to lower her high blood pressure. She says she feels like a guinea pig, first because *she's* never tried it before and also because it's only been available for a few years. But she's not a test subject. Thousands of people before her took the drug over long periods before it was approved. The odds of something awful happening *this* time are pretty remote.

That's not to say that strange things don't ever happen with medicines. They do. There is no guarantee Mary won't have a side-effect that requires changing to another drug or one that could even hurt her. It's a matter of weighing the odds based on hard science and statistical results. If the drug has been effective for thousands of patients with no unexpected safety issues and with manageable side-effects, the odds are very much in Mary's favor. But it's never a sure bet.

Nothing about treating the human body can be guaranteed. Life *is* risk. And virtually everything we do and a great many things we don't do are a gamble. You have to weigh the odds.

Mary faces a far greater risk if she does not take a drug to control her high blood pressure. She may find this difficult to appreciate when she's fighting the anxiety of starting a prescription medication. I can sympathize with her distress.

I know flying is much safer than traveling a long distance by car. I know the statistics, the facts, and the scientific evidence that demonstrate jumbo jets can, and almost always do, land safely. But it still *feels* like a huge risk. I wrestle with an anxious, hand-wringing little voice until that monstrous machine is back on the ground. Climbing into my familiar car for a road trip would feel much more comfortable.

If I need to get to New York from Oregon, I fly. Logic drowns out the frightened voice. I give greater weight to what I know than what I fear. No guarantees, of course, just really good odds.

I greatly value the non-scientific aspects of our life and culture. Spirituality, emotional well-being, and artistic expression are important factors in sustaining good health. But we should embrace science and technology in the same way, not as a likely threat but as a potential life preserver.

Meditation, energy healing, and living "by intention" can enhance the quality of our lives, but they won't fly us around the globe, enable us to make an emergency phone call, or identify a small cancer when it's still curable. Science and technology do that, and only as the result of a long and rigorous process that really works. No arm waving. No philosophizing. Just hard-earned results.

They are essential tools for enhancing and preserving human life, although we often take them for granted. Who today celebrates that smallpox and polio are no longer rampant; that pneumonia can now be cured; that the average lifespan is no longer 40 years; or that deadly bacterial infections are less deadly? We are all guilty of a "So, what's next?" attitude.

My CD player stops functioning on a long drive. I'm indignant. "Damn thing!" Yet during the last six years when it worked perfectly, did it occur to me to appreciate hearing music and books and lectures from the world's finest minds, all stored on shiny little disks that didn't even exist before 1982?

Acting like a spoiled brat as I take my amazing toys for granted is one thing. But forgetting, and thereby dismissing, life before antibiotics, MRI imaging, vaccines, and chemotherapy is quite another. Every day, I see patients with a health problem or disease that would have killed them a few generations ago, back when people were ecstatic to live to be 60.

Consider two endings to this story. An eight-year-old girl gets a flu that develops into pneumonia. She dies. Her younger brother, sister, and parents are devastated. The father copes with the loss by drinking too much. He withdraws from his family and friends. The mother stoically goes through the motions devoid of joy. Before long, the parents divorce introducing the two remaining children to another nightmare. Few tragedies have such deep and broad repercussions as the loss of a child.

Or, this: The girl lives because she is treated with a brand new chemical, an antibiotic. She survives to live a full life, remaining close to her siblings and parents, eventually arranging their 50th wedding anniversary party.

It's easy to imagine ourselves in the shoes of someone hit by tragedy. The ripple effects of a tragedy *avoided* are harder to appreciate. But they're out there.

A father is on hand to high-five his son after a little league game; he did not die in his 40s of a heart attack the way *his* father had. A couple enjoys pride and happiness in the achievements of their child, the one who survived that annoying bout with pneumonia back when she was eight.

The Dark Side of Modern Medicine

There always is one. Medications can backfire to annoy, injure or even kill the person they were supposed to help. People can die from complications of routine surgery. But side-effects are mostly reversible and death-by-treatment is very rare.

There is actually a more serious dark side, and it would be dishonest not to address it. The miracle antibiotics that saved millions of lives and kicked infection off the top ten causes of death are losing their effectiveness in today's world. New breeds of germs have evolved, the kind that eat penicillin for lunch.

Decades ago, a rare, mutant bacteria, might be directed by its damaged code to produce some altered enzyme at a furious pace all day long. This diversion of energy meant that it grew more slowly than its hundred trillion family members. Enter Penicillin. The entire "normal" family is wiped out, but not our mutant bug. His timing was perfect. The abundant new enzyme he can't stop making turned out to neutralize the effects of the antibiotic. Our mutant continues to breed, producing drug-resistant offspring.

Scientists thought that by withholding use of a particular antibiotic for a while, the regular, non-resistant germs would return, again multiply faster than the mutant bugs, thus replacing them and restoring the original balance.

This was how it worked when I was in college. I actually did these experiments. But, unlike me, microorganisms have gotten much smarter since I graduated. Now, they don't waste any extra energy developing resistant proteins *until* they encounter the antibiotic attacking them. So they don't let their weaker cousins evict them.

What's worse, completely unrelated species of bacteria now have the ability to communicate with each other in a chilling way. A super-bug can share its most resistant genes with a different type of bug by passing a DNA "plasmid" through its membrane into the cell of its apprentice, bestowing the same resistance properties.

The result is a steadily rising percentage of deadly drug-resistant infections. They thrive in places *bathed* in antibiotics: our hospitals, convalescent facilities, and nursing homes. These super-germs are like hardened criminals after decades of prison time. They're tough, they're mean, but unlike criminals, we have no way to contain them.

Sounds like the Sci-Fi movie of the week, right? Except it's not fiction. It's ecology. We've taken our science and unleashed it on the planet's other inhabitants. And in *this* form of germ warfare, the germs are fighting back.

We have fared better in our fight against virus infections. Vaccinations have worked out well, in part because viruses are not living organisms. They are bits of protein-covered genetic stuff that can program an innocent living cell to make more viruses.

A good example is a floppy disk compared to a working computer. The disk doesn't have motors, lights, or busy silicon chips like a computer. It can lay dormant in a drawer for years without the need for electricity to keep its program intact. But if the data on that inert little disk is toxic, should it find its way into your floppy disk drive, it can infect your computer, ordering it to copy and spread the virus code all over the Internet, then command your machine to self-destruct. A "computer virus" is an excellent analogy to the way a virus behaves in real life.

A vaccination gives our bodies a tiny exposure to these viral proteins. This triggers the production of antibodies which then coat any newly-made viruses before they can attach to our cells to trick them into making more virus copies. Vaccinations have been wonderful. There's only a tiny amount of smallpox virus left on the planet for the various militaries in the world to play with.

The Western Hemisphere was certified as free from poliovirus in 1994, an accomplishment achieved through the Oral Polio Vaccine. And since 1980, the incidence of polio in the rest of the world has dropped over 80 percent.

There is a small risk associated with the Polio Vaccine. Between 1973 and 1984, there were 105 cases of vaccine-associated poliomyelitis (the paralyzing form of the disease) reported in the United States. This translates into one case for every 2.6 million doses distributed. In the decades prior to vaccination, the incidence of poliomyelitis ranged from twenty to fifty *thousand* new cases each year. Just do the math.

Viruses, like bacteria, can mutate. This happens both randomly and in response to selective pressure from antiviral drugs. It makes sense. Alterations to the viral code can occur as the hijacked cell copies it over and over again. In fact, some viruses have genes that promote their own mutation. The only viruses that manage to get themselves successfully reproduced in an otherwise "immune" person are mutants that escape our antibodies or our drugs; their mutation makes them "invisible" to our protective systems.

All this might inspire you to ask: Would we have been better off had antibiotics and vaccines never been developed in the first place?

Before we had antibiotics to destroy lethal bacteria, people had only their own immune systems to determine if they lived or died from an infection. If their bodies became overwhelmed (septic) from pneumonia or an infected wound, they died. If their immune systems prevailed, they recovered. The son of President Calvin Coolidge died in the White House of "blood poisoning" caused by a foot blister he developed playing tennis. All the power of the Presidency could do nothing to save the young man.

Things changed dramatically with the discovery of penicillin and the creation of other antibiotics. In the future, if we find ourselves without any effective antibiotics, one could make the argument that we had a century of considerable well-being, and then Mother Nature stepped back in. Would you say the world is worse for having had a hundred years of effective antibiotics treatment?

It's not as if dying from these new germs is different than dying from the old ones. Dead is dead. Is it better to have never had something than to have had and lost it? Not in my case, and probably not in yours. Before I was ever conceived, my mother's appendicitis had to be treated with surgery *and* antibiotics to save her life. I'm really happy to be here.

I don't believe we'll revert to being powerless against infection, but what I *believe* doesn't count. Only time will tell. We will hear a great deal about this problem in the years to come. Until a solution emerges, doctors must curb unnecessary antibiotic use. No small challenge for hospitals where delaying antibiotics is a major cause of death. The widespread use of antibiotics in the feed of poultry and livestock is another dangerous practice that needs to be seriously reconsidered.

However, for most of us, antibiotic use to treat a child with pneumonia or deadly spinal meningitis is a no-brainer. So are treatments for other reasons, like prescribing pain medication to someone suffer-ing from injury or surgical pain or the process of dying.

The choice to treat becomes less obvious, however, when decid-ing whether to take a drug to lower one's cholesterol or blood pressure or to treat one's mood or stress level. The more abstract the reason for taking medication, the easier it is to focus only on the risk, thereby sidestepping a *balanced* evaluation of risk, side-effects, *and* benefits. And sometimes, the way it's all presented to the patient doesn't help either.

Let's say your cholesterol has been on the high side for two blood tests in a row. The doctor says it's running 295 and your LDL portion is a whopping 202, so he wants you to take medication to lower it. This, he says, will reduce your risk for a heart attack. It will also set you back about $80 per month and could make your muscles hurt for no apparent reason. You must return for a blood test in six weeks to see if it's working and to make sure it's not damaging your liver. *"Okay, see you in six weeks…oh, did you have a question?"*

"Uh…*yeah*! *Liver* damage? Liver *damage*? You want me to pay a thousand bucks a year to poison my liver? Because I *might, maybe, possibly, some day* have a heart attack? Hey, doc, I feel f-i-n-e. Never better, in fact. And what the hell is an LDL portion?"

After reluctantly taking his hand off the doorknob and turning back, the doctor might explain that the risk of liver damage is infini-tesimally small, that muscle pain is much more common, but reversible. He may add that you don't *have* to take the medicine; you *could* try a low-fat diet and exercise program if you're worried about taking a drug. But mainly, he seems confused by your protests. He thinks what needs to be done is obvious. And it is…to scientists and other doctors.

What's going on inside the head of the person in the white coat scribbling an illegible prescription for an expensive bottle of pills? Why does he or she expect you to swallow a pill every day forever or at least for the foreseeable future? You're paying good money, one way or another, for his recommendation, so you are entitled to some an-swers. He may be rushing to the bottom line because there are 10 patients still in the waiting room and its 4:00 p.m., but the most likely explanation is this: he's playing the odds—on your behalf. And he knows your odds are better if you take the drug than if you don't.

Most of us would rather fancy our physician as a well-adjusted provider of wisdom and solutions than as a high-rolling gambler in need of a twelve-step program. Throwing dice with our lives is not a comforting image. Shouldn't risking liver damage warrant a sit-down? And what about our famous Oath: "Physician, first do no harm"?

Physicians are sometimes accused of disregarding this part of the Hippocratic Oath. I've heard or read the echo of that admonishment from many new-age alternative medicine gurus, often when promoting their own services and exclusive line of *all-natural* remedies. The suggestion is that doctors throw drugs or vaccinations at patients willy-nilly, indifferent to who gets hurt and who gets helped.

And this opinion is not limited to health practitioners with viewpoints that oppose mine. Many people, including some doctors, take this quote to mean that if there is any chance for a treatment to hurt a patient, then we should use it only as a last resort. This turns out to be a very dangerous idea.

Hippocrates was not appealing to physicians to avoid all risk. If he was, he'd be telling physicians to quit their jobs altogether. Risk itself isn't the issue. Risk is *absolutely unavoidable.* Trying to avoid risk is foolish. Taking action in any direction is a risk. Doing nothing is a risk. The only way to deal with risk is to understand it and then *manage* it.

If you call me for an appointment because a headache won't go away, I'll look at my schedule and probably sigh. But, because I'm a nice guy who sympathizes with persistent headaches, I'll tell you to come in around noon and to please bring a book or magazine. BAM! I just put you at risk. People with headaches bad enough to call me probably shouldn't be driving. Headaches make people a bit stupid; the blood flow to their brain is actually altered, and testing has shown that they just aren't all there.

So, should you crash your car on your drive to my office, it may well be my fault. In fact, this would be a perfect situation for a house call.

Let's say you get to the office without incident. You now have to endure the dreaded waiting room where every magazine has been touched by sick patients. Maybe you'll pick up an infection; hopefully, not one that's resistant to antibiotics. If I interpreted the words *Physician, first do no harm* literally, I wouldn't let you into my waiting room. It could mean doing you harm. I'd be doing harm, also, if I told you to stay home, take two aspirin, and call me in the morning. The headache might be from meningitis or bleeding in your skull from an aneurysm and you wouldn't last the night. Drat! Cornered like a rat. Either way, I've betrayed my sacred oath.

Actually, I never made that particular promise. What a relief! I *did* take the Oath of Hippocrates, but it turns out "…first do no harm" isn't part of it. It's a common misconception since the quote is attributed to the same great man. Regardless, this absurd exercise demonstrates how doctors, like everyone else, cause risks no matter what they do or *don't do*.

Let's go back to our problem with high cholesterol and get a second opinion. Our new doctor is more concerned about the side-effects of the medication, knows how expensive it is, and wants to do his part to reduce healthcare costs. He prefers a conservative approach, so he encourages you to restrict the fat in your diet and work out three times a week. He tells you to come back in a few months to check your cholesterol.

This physician sets in motion a different set of risks. You could suffer a heart attack or stroke in those next few months, a disaster that might have been avoided with medication. You might fail to stick to your diet-exercise regimen. Next thing you know you're saying, "To hell with it; if he didn't think I needed a drug right now, my risk of a heart attack must not be too bad." Chances are you'll skip that follow-up appointment, so doctor number two could lose the opportunity to prescribe the medication at a later date. His concern about healthcare costs isn't anything to cheer about either. The cost of a lifetime of medication is a drop in the bucket compared to emergency heart surgery and rehabilitative therapy, or the cost of your life.

The presence of risk is a given. The doctor's job is to identify and help you actively manage it. Sometimes the greatest harm done by a physician is through *inaction*.

People have high expectations of their physicians and expect them to cover all the bases: to look for everything, find every findable problem, and keep them alive. Most physicians do their best. Some, unfortunately, work hard to stay in their comfort zone, avoiding all but the most conservative measures.

They do so for good reason. They may get blamed, sued, and professionally broken if unexpected reactions to treatment hurt their patient. Yet, they will never *ever* get the credit for preventing a heart attack or stroke. Mathematics states that you cannot prove a negative, meaning that we never get to know which patients escaped the heart attack or stroke they would have had, thanks to preventive intervention.

So which doctor is right? The one who's quick to prescribe a drug and doesn't seem to care about killing your liver? Or the other, who has faith in you to "get healthy" and is willing to let you die trying? Of course, we can't know the answer until we know which choice gives you the best *odds* of living a longer, healthier life.

Whatever those odds turn out to be, understand this: neither doctor knows your future. No one, not your physician, your minister, your parents, not even your astrologer can tell you whether you are going to have a heart attack, a stroke, or if you'll develop a certain cancer. In fact, to say that your doctor gave you a "clean bill of health" implies knowledge that simply doesn't exist. But, we *can* estimate the odds of these things occurring. And when you make a change, such as taking a medicine or altering a habit, we can re-estimate those odds.

To understand the difference between fortune-telling and an educated understanding of the odds, consider this: I can't tell you if a penny you toss will come up heads or tails, but we both know the odds for heads is 50 percent, the odds for tails is 50 percent. If you toss the coin many times and record the results of "heads" and "tails," you'll get about an equal number in the two columns. The more you toss the coin, the closer the percentage will be to 50-50.

Most of us know that when flipping a coin, aside from superstition or personal preference, it doesn't really matter whether we choose heads or tails. Likewise, if a doctor can choose between two equally beneficial treatments with the same potential side-effects, he could just flip a coin. And it would be fine if he had a personal preference for one over another. It would be fine if he was superstitious about blue pills and always recommended the green. Either way, his judgment would be okay *in this case.* But I probably don't have to tell you that "six of one, half a dozen of the other" very rarely happens. Treatment options almost always come with a wide range of potential benefits, side-effects and risks. We just have to do the math.

Most of our knowledge in medicine comes to us as statistics about very large groups of people. One good type of knowledge is based on two large groups of research volunteers who participate in a study that lasts for years. One group gets Treatment A. The other group gets Treatment B to see which treatment gets better results. Sometimes, one of the two treatments is actually a placebo. This will be a "double-blind" study if no one, neither volunteers nor the study personnel, knows which person is getting which treatment until the program ends. This is also a "prospective" study, because a specific question is asked in advance, and the entire study is designed to answer that one question. These studies are of great value to physicians.

There are also "retrospective" studies, so named because a question is asked *after* a body of data has been collected; we look back in time for our answer. These are cheaper, easier and, therefore, more numerous. Results from this kind of research are often cited and can affect our clinical practice as well. This is not such a good thing, because they are far less valuable than prospective studies.

Here's how they work. One might use, say, a hospital computer to review five years of charts to identify patients who received the cholesterol-lowering drugs, Zocor and Lipitor. We ask some questions.

How many of these patients made it home from the hospital alive?— trying to get a feel if one is better at saving lives than the other.

What were the average cholesterols for each group?—trying to learn if one drug is stronger than the other.

Did one group complain of more muscle pain or have more abnormal liver tests than the other?—trying to get a feel if one is safer than the other.

They could track down the actual patients to see how they're doing now, long after their stay in the hospital. How many have since passed away, how many went on to become diabetic or to need heart bypass surgery, etc? It seems like an abundant gift basket of information that we can explore to further our knowledge. But like most gift baskets, looks can be deceiving—very attractive on the outside, not so valuable when you look deeper.

The value of a study depends on our ability to assign a true cause and effect to the treatment being considered. For example, the Atkins diet, a weight loss fad that was very popular a few years ago, was structured around eating very few carbohydrates, starches and sweets, while chowing down on lots of fat and protein. If we want to know if the high-fat Atkins diet causes heart attacks, we could design a prospective study, the good kind, where one large group is given a normal control diet and the other an Atkins diet. We would follow thousands of people for the years it would take to answer our question: which group has more heart attacks?

After all that work, it would be devastating to learn that the designers of the study, after carefully matching the two research groups for age, gender and many other traits, forgot to ask participants about diabetes. Unless the same number of diabetics just happened to be assigned to the Atkins group and the control group, you may as well throw the entire study away.

If one group had even 5 percent more diabetics than the other, the information about heart attacks could be useless, because diabetes gives a person a huge risk for heart disease and is likely to swamp out any effect, good or bad, from the diet. It's hard to notice a ripple at the beach when a tidal wave is crashing down in the same place!

If I were to design such a study, I might exclude all people who had diabetes. This way, there would be fewer overall heart attacks but each one would have a higher chance of being due to diet. Eventually, I could see if there was a heart risk to the Atkins diet. Sounds good. Maybe I'll teach the world something valuable when I publish the results.

But there is also a down side to leaving diabetics out of my study. Many of the people who turned to Atkins were overweight diabetics. If I excluded diabetics, even if my Atkins patients were dying faster than the control group, I would have to say something like this: "When compared to our control diet, *non-diabetic* people demonstrated an 8.5 percent greater risk of heart attack when eating the Atkins diet than when eating our control diet."

First, a quick reality check: I know of no good studies that *ever* suggested the Atkins Diet causes heart attacks. People may assume it does, because it contains a lot of fat. But people lose weight on it too. And few things matter more to the health of an obese diabetic than weight loss. So even if I actually did my big study and used the results to sell my own new "South Bend Diet," I had better be darn careful about the claims I make. Atkins might actually save the lives of some diabetics even if it adds a risk to the lives of thin, non-diabetics. Once again, there is *no evidence* that it does either! Who we let in and keep out of our studies has a huge effect in correctly interpreting the results!

What about our *retrospective* hospital review? We may compare the fates of patients who happened to be on one of our two cholesterol-lowering medications, but transforming such data into useful cholesterol-related advice for my office patients would be completely impossible and meaningless. The people studied through the hospital records in no way represent an average population. Here are just a few of the reasons.

First, our study reviews records at a single hospital. Since the patients all wound up in the same hospital, with rare exception, they will be from the same area of the country. Health issues vary widely throughout the country, and, unless I live and practice in the same area, the results may have no bearing on my patient population.

Second, all these people had serious health problems or they wouldn't have been hospitalized. Any deaths, muscle aches, or liver problems in a hospital are probably related to their illness and are unlikely to be due to a single little drug that they've probably been taking for years.

Third, the patients are likely to be older, poorer, more prone to mental illness, and more likely to have unhealthy habits such as smoking, excessive drinking, or other drug use than the average population. It's just a reality of our hospital populations.

Finally, the two groups taking either Zocor or Lipitor will not be equally matched in terms of age, gender, general health status, percentage of smokers, diabetics, etc. When research comparisons are not based on factors that are specific and balanced, the resulting data is not an apples-to-apples comparison; it's more like apples to bonbons, having little or no relevance or value.

So I could not apply the results of that retrospective study to the patients I see. The impact of two medications is mixed with the much more dramatic impact of being in the hospital in the first place. This information is useless to me. But it's the kind of study that salesmen and the media typically quote.

We must use large-scale, well-controlled, *prospective* studies by reputable research institutions to make sound treatment recommendations for patients.

Why bother to do retrospective studies at all? The example of our fictitious hospital study is deliberately dreadful in order to point out inherent problems with retrospective study design itself. Some useful information can be obtained, but the best use of retrospective data is to help us search for clues. If our review uncovered a significant, unexpected difference in outcomes between the two groups, it would support the need for a *prospective* study for determining if one drug was truly better than the other.

A real-life example of this is right now being reported in the medical news, and it's forcing me to change some long-held beliefs. Personally, I hate when that happens. But, as a scientist and physician, I welcome it with enthusiasm.

For almost a decade we have been advising heart patients to take high doses of the vitamin folic acid, also called folate. The logic was this: several *retrospective analyses* of large groups of patients showed that people with elevated blood levels of a substance call "homocysteine" had more heart attacks than people with normal or low levels.

Taking folic acid lowers homocysteine levels, especially when mixed with vitamin B6. As a result, we've been measuring homocysteine levels for years and prescribing folic acid when levels are elevated. Heck, insurance companies even pay for the blood test and for prescription-strength folic acid when needed.

We also know, incidentally, that folic acid supplements prevent certain birth defects when given to pregnant women. It must be good for us!

Then several prospective studies got underway, specifically designed to prove whether or not folic acid has a beneficial effect. Several small studies have shown no effect at all, and now one very recent, very large, and, apparently, well-conducted study from Norway found that not only did folic acid treatment fail to prevent heart attacks, combining it with vitamin B6 seems to make a heart attack more likely!

Folic acid may be great for preventing spina bifida in newborns, but if you're Norwegian with characteristics similar to the patients in their study, taking it with B6 to prevent a heart attack may be a bad idea.

We don't even know for sure if a high level of homocysteine is a bad thing. The retrospective observations of homocysteine and heart disease merely suggested an *association*, not a direct cause and effect. Perhaps some other process causes heart disease and just happens to raise homocysteine levels as an incidental side-effect. If that's true, prescribing folic acid would be like trying to reduce a child's fever by taking some of the mercury out of the thermometer.

As I write, the folic acid issue remains unresolved. For the moment, I will be recommending folic acid as an option for patients with known heart disease and a high homocysteine level. But I will instruct them not to take it with vitamin B6 until we learn more. Perhaps by the time you read this, I will be recommending something slightly different based on the latest information available.

What, then, do we do with reliable, applicable information when we get it? We've learned that diabetics live longer if we put them on a cholesterol-lowering drug of the statin class, *regardless* of their actual cholesterol levels. Strange but true. What should a diabetic and her doctor do with this information? After all, Lipitor or Zocor might kill her too. How should she make her choice to use or reject the drug?

To gain some insight into how physicians approach these questions, let's use an analogy. Imagine for a moment that everyone on the planet lived in houses of ten residents each. Unfortunately, each house is haunted by its own ghost, the kind that can cause heart attacks. All the ghosts are menacing but some are active, others are taking long naps. Every now and then, an occupant dies suddenly of a heart attack. No one, not even the ghosts, know who will die or when. But what is certain is that those in House A have a long-established history of losing five out of ten people every ten years whereas House B only loses about two out of ten in the same period.

I am your doctor. I have one trick up my sleeve. I can move you from House A to House B. That's all. I have no way of knowing if you will be one of the five who will be doomed if you stay in the first house or one of the two in the other house.

You may survive in either house, you may suffer a fatal heart attack in either house, but we only know the odds: 20 percent chance of dying if you move compared to a 50 percent chance if you stay put.

By the way, relocating will increase your rent about $80 per month. There's a one-in-a-million chance that you could die in an accident during the move and a 2 percent chance you'll have an allergic reaction to the new house, forcing you to move back to House A briefly until we find a safer residence. So what would your decision be?

It's not a trick question. If you have to think about it you're making it too complicated, or maybe you have a death wish. The odds would be overwhelmingly in your favor if you started packing.

This is an abbreviated example of how doctors decide, statistically, what's best for their patients. We cannot make conclusive predictions about the future health of any patient. It's an *educated* flip of the coin. We simply know that reducing the risk factors for all our patients will prevent many of them from having a heart attack, stroke, or other medical disaster. Yes, we're playing the odds, but unlike Las Vegas, we stick with the ones in our favor.

So is all this betting a form of science? You bet. In medicine, applied science is as much about knowing the odds as it is about complicated biology, physiology, and chemistry. And for many, the odds for a longer, healthier life can be increased by taking medication.

To avoid any dangerous misunderstanding, I must point out a crucial difference between medical gambling and trying to beat the house in Vegas. They're distinct in a fundamental way. When you apply the rules of Las Vegas gambling to a game like roulette, you stand the chance of winning *much more* than your bet. For example, if you bet on number 18, the odds of the ball landing on that number are 38-to-1. If you win, you'll get back your bet *plus* 35 times that amount. This is why people risk losing again and again—the lure of a big payoff.

Playing the odds in medicine is radically different. There are no 36-to-1 winners. The game of health or illness is not a *winner-gets-rich* but rather a *loser-gets-hurt* game, so it's foolish to bet on anything but the most likely winner.

Whatever we do or don't do is a gamble. It's not about winning more than you have. You are already alive and you own your current state of health. The game is how best to protect what you already own. And we don't have the option of not playing.

If you apply the rules of medical gambling to our example of roulette, it goes something like this:

▶ **You must play. If you win, you live. If you lose, you die.**

▶ **You only get to roll once.**

▶ **You can bet that the ball *will* land on 18 OR you can bet that it *won't* land on 18.**

Betting against 18 gives you odds of 37 out of 38, more than a 97 percent chance that you'll live. If you bet on 18, the odds are only 1 in 38, or less than 3 percent chance of survival.

Many would agree that someone who gets only one bet in the game of life and chooses the long shot, even though they stand to win nothing extra for all the added risk, is probably too dumb to live anyway. Guess what? That's exactly what many not-so-dumb people are doing right now. They accept needless threats to their lives by ignoring them and turning their backs on simple, safe, and effective ways to reduce those threats. We invite risk by failing to recognize it. Or, when we do discover it, we do nothing about it. High blood pressure. An abnormal mole. A family history of breast, ovarian, or colon cancer. And we don't take the next step to fix the problem.

Of course, there are times when playing the odds smartly doesn't pay off. It's rare but it happens. Someone in their 50s who makes every effort to lower their risks still suffers a heart attack. We may also know a hard-living, overweight, diabetic, chain smoker who dies peacefully at 95.

"Look Doc, my friend's grandfather enjoyed 2 packs of unfiltered Camels every day of his life and lived to be 90. I figure the crap about smoking is just scare tactics."

I heard there's a guy who actually won the lottery *twice,* but I'm not about to abandon my job and bet every dollar I own on Powerball tickets.

All these situations, the patient who does everything right and things turn out all wrong, the chain-smoking centenarian, and the double lottery winner are very, very, very long shots. Betting on such outcomes for yourself would be foolish.

So if managing risk is equivalent to accepting that your favorite number *isn't* likely to come up in one play at the roulette table, how do you then chart a course of action?

The media gives you hype, half-truths, and partial facts. The scientific research, which may or may not apply to you, is massive, complex, and may as well be written in ancient Greek for most of us. How do you know what is most likely to add years to your life?

Part 2 of this book was written to be an introduction to the world of reliable information and sound advice. And, if you've read this far in Part 1, congratulations! You will be better able to read what follows with a critical mind, to pick and choose what advice applies to your life and what doesn't. That's a handy skill. Taking control and learning what you need to manage your own health will be a very freeing experience.

Keep in mind that what is known today may be out of date tomorrow, so you are undertaking a life-long process of staying informed and actively participating in your plan of care. This book started becoming obsolete before it ever reached you. My website at **www.stupidreasonspeopledie.com** is there to help you with updates and corrections. Yes, in medicine there are always corrections.

Another reliable source of information should be your own doctor. "Yeah, right," some of you are mumbling. I've heard the stories of frustration.

"He didn't answer my question."

"She explained it, kind of. She was gone before I could process what she said and ask for clarification."

"He never returned my call."

It would be great if all doctors were good communicators and competent scientists with plenty of time on their hands. Fact is, they're only human, and nobody is good at all things.

Usually, the problem is not an unwillingness to share information but a basic difference between the way patients and physicians view the world of science and health. Believe it or not, you are already in a better position to understand your doctor on his or her own terms. Now, I hope to make it even easier.

Say what you want about big-science medicine, but office physicians on the frontlines of patient care simply have no motive to give advice that is skewed. The only thing they're "selling" is preserving or restoring your health. They don't make a dime prescribing expensive medication. In fact, doctors can actually be financially penalized for doing so.

Most of us don't sell supplements or other extra services to add to our income. More and more, our license to practice medicine is held to a standard called "outcome-based medicine." Basically, this means we get in trouble if we fail to do certain things that are widely considered effective.

For example, if a diabetic is leaking protein in their urine but their physician fails to test for it, find it, and treat it during their annual visit, that doctor is considered guilty of malpractice.

As much as I enjoy making fun of our media, real news can sometimes be delivered with a health-scare story. When the news relates to your health and treatment, this should be the springboard for a conversation with your doctor. He or she has no motivation to conceal or alter the facts and knows that a patient armed with the facts is more likely to participate constructively in the plan of care.

What are the questions to ask?

Your doctor makes some recommendation, such as starting a new medication, having a CAT scan or stress ECG, "waiting and watching" to monitor for elevations in your blood pressure, or even rushing you to the hospital for urgent testing. You are no longer passive, but though you want to know more, it may be hard to know where to begin. Here are some suggestions.

How serious is the existing or potential problem?

You want to know if this *is* a big deal, *might* be a big deal, or is just a minor precaution. Let's say for the past three days you have chest pain and sweat heavily *every* time you climb stairs. Prior to three days ago it had only happened a few times over several months. This could be a VERY BIG DEAL. Your doctor would want you in the hospital to have a cardiologist perform an angiogram of your coronary arteries. It is likely one or more of the arteries will need to be re-opened.

Another patient might experience pain in his left arm every time he sleeps on it. He rushes to his doctor, knowing it might be a sign of a heart attack. He's worried. The doctor can reproduce his exact pain by pushing the shoulder into a certain position, indicating the pain is caused by inflammation in his shoulder, not his heart. Thankfully, it's not a life or death situation, but immediate attention may help to prevent further injury. His doctor suggests an anti-inflammatory medication and physical therapy to help the inflamed shoulder to heal.

What are the consequences if I do nothing?
How likely is it I will face those consequences?

For you, the patient with chest pain, the price of doing nothing could be death or a major heart attack that kills a chunk of the heart. The likelihood of these consequences is high, about 10 percent within the next few weeks, 50 percent within a year. There is also the risk that doing nothing would make it impossible for you to walk 20 feet, forget trying to climb stairs. You could pass out, breaking your neck or something else when you fall.

For the guy with the sore shoulder, doing nothing might lead to further damage requiring surgery, especially if he continues to use it in his physical activities. A swollen "rotator cuff" can tear if overused.

Are there alternatives to the treatment being recommended?
Would they be just as effective?
What is the downside of the alternative?

In our case of chest pain or "unstable angina," there are no medically accepted alternatives to an angiogram, although new technology may be available to determine what is going on in the coronary arteries without threading a catheter into the heart. The bottom line is we must look for the partial blockage likely to be causing the symptoms. If it's there, we must fix it. Not much leeway here.

On the other hand, a sore shoulder can often be treated by a number of alternatives to medication that might work as well or even better. Patients who choose to try chiropractic treatment, acupuncture, or other approaches may have great results. The very worst outcome: they wind up needing surgery.

How effective is the treatment being considered?

Will an angiogram and likely placement of a stent to keep the coronary artery open lower your risk of a heart attack? For how long? Then what? How long is recovery after the procedure? How long before I'll be able to climb stairs, jog, have sex?

The answers to these questions may surprise you. The procedure can make you feel like a kid again. Angina of this type usually comes on slowly; patients have often subconsciously accepted a gradual loss of stamina and physical ability as the natural process of getting old.

When the blood flows more freely again, you may feel great. On the other hand, the stent alone may not prolong life. The process of coronary disease will continue unless it is halted with medication. If that doesn't happen, the big heart attack is still ahead.

Treating a sore shoulder with ibuprofen and physical therapy may be only slightly more effective than doing nothing. Resting the shoulder without allowing it to freeze up from lack of movement is what really matters. So if I had to miss work three days a week for a month to keep my physical therapy appointments, I might choose to forego that advice and keep my vacation time intact.

What are the direct risks of the treatment being considered? How dangerous are they and how common are they?

I've left the most commonly asked question for last, because I want to emphasize: it is not necessarily the most important one. Focusing on the risks of taking action, undergoing surgery, or starting a medication, blocks us from carefully considering our whole situation. Ask the other four questions first. Once *their* answers are well understood, the direct risk of an intervention will be seen in perspective to the big picture. This is a very handy point of view.

The most serious risks of an angiogram and stent placement include:

> The procedure could cause damage to the very artery the cardiologist is trying to open, and you could find yourself waking up from emergency surgery to repair it. In other words, there's a possibility of open heart bypass surgery.

> The procedure could itself lead to a heart attack if a branch of the heart's blood supply got completely blocked and could not be re-opened in time. This is very rare.

> The puncture wound for the procedure could bleed a lot or become infected.

We could go on down the list all the way to having nightmares or the quarter-inch scar in your groin from the catheter, but in a big-stakes game like unstable heart disease these lose importance.

Emergency surgery during an angiogram is serious and people can die in the process. *But it is rare.* In the past 20 years, I know of one patient out of hundreds who needed the emergency surgery, and he didn't die. Other complications can occur but are far less serious.

An extra day in the hospital to make sure the bleeding stops or going home after the procedure with an antibiotic prescription are the more common "complications."

Our sore shoulder patient? It could actually feel worse with physical therapy, and, in my experience, this happens about 10 percent to 20 percent of the time. Medication like ibuprofen can cause stomach upset and bleeding ulcers. I once prescribed this treatment for my former little league coach, and he wound up in the hospital with a dangerous bleeding ulcer. I think I might have felt worse than he did.

Let's get back to our patient with the cholesterol of 295 and the low-density lipoprotein complex (LDL) portion of 202. That was actually me. It was 1993, I was 38 years old with two small children, and I needed answers. I studied what was known at that time about guys like me with the same cholesterol problem. I took into account other things like my blood pressure, non-smoker status, and family history. I discovered that my high cholesterol was one thing, but the high LDL portion was the bigger problem. LDL is the so-called "bad cholesterol." Good and bad cholesterol are more about the vehicle in which cholesterol travels than the stuff itself. I have the kind of vehicles that could make a mess out of arteries.

It seemed to happen overnight. Two years earlier, my numbers were something to brag about. I re-checked several times over the next few months and the results only got worse. Damn. I was turning into my father!

This was just about the time that the first survival studies were being published about two cholesterol-lowering drugs, Zocor and Pravachol, and the results looked good. Although my weight was normal and I was in good shape, I tried the jogging and eating the rabbit food bit for a while with no improvement. So I chose to try Zocor.

I've been on it ever since with one or two periods of time when I just had to see what would happen without it. It's always the same. On the drug, my cholesterol is the envy of any 20-year-old; off it, I break some of my own office records for lousy lab results.

I must add here that I'm not just treating numbers on a lab printout. Managing heart risk has become much more sophisticated since 1993, and I've kept up. I now live in a "haunted house" where only one person dies every 25 years. I plan to be there to walk my beautiful daughter down the aisle and to wrestle with my son's kids as I did with him. Science, technology, and my ability to understand and interpret them will help me do it.

Coming up in Part 2, we'll talk about the screening tests and treatments that are most likely to extend your life. Armed with an open mind and good data, you can approach your doctor with a list of your requirements, which he or she will authorize and order. Yeah, Right.

One day, that might be the case. But not today. There is one more hurdle to get past before you can really put state-of-the-art information and technology to work for you and your loved ones.

The health insurance system in this country is designed to offer a level of service called the *standard of care*. This is a level based on the past, typically five or ten years behind the state-of-the-art in technology and knowledge. Our system will not provide coverage for the most current advances in screening or treatment. Nor should it.

It doesn't matter how much a person pays for health insurance or if someone has paid into Medicare for 50 years, true state-of-the-art prevention will *never* come from a middle man. Until we can get past the idea that our insurance or government healthcare plan *should* offer us what we want, we will never be free to get the care we need.

It is simply not possible for our healthcare delivery system, in its present form, to provide excellence in preventive health.

BROKEN BUREAUCRACY

"How would you feel if your car insurance company started telling you which gas you must buy and when you could and couldn't buy it, which mechanics you could use and whether or not you deserved roadside service?

Chapter 8

What Do You Mean My Insurance Won't Pay For It?

Doesn't it make you furious when you pay hundreds of dollars a month for a health insurance plan, which then spends most of its efforts trying to avoid paying for your care? Maybe you've paid into the Medicare fund with your taxes for decades, and now they are refusing to pay for anything *they* deem "not medically necessary."

If you've ever had the experience of getting a healthcare claim denied, this couple's conversation from my own medical practice might resonate with you:

"Doc, our insurance refuses to pay for so many important things. Our last doctor recommended we each get complete physicals. So we got them, and our insurance hardly paid for any of it because they said it was 'preventive.' We paid those jerks over four hundred bucks a month for years."

"Last year we went on Medicare and found that they won't pay for anything unless *they* think it's 'medically necessary.' They don't think that includes annual physicals but we believe it does, and so did our last doctor. Yet when I asked him to put something in the bill to show it is 'medically necessary,' he said he couldn't. So we had to pay at both ends. That's why we changed to you. Will you *please* put down something on the bill to make them pay?"

To have to beg or even change doctors to get coverage for preventive medicine is outrageous. Vital medical services that affect our very lives are being denied by health insurance, by Medicare and, of course, by those wretched HMOs. It's become a desperate game, trying to trick them into paying for what we deserve and truly need.

They are literally *killing* some of us by denying us adequate preventive care.

What should we do to correct this problem and protect ourselves? Here is the list of proactive steps I actually give to my patients. Following the steps on this list will remove the biggest barrier to receiving the latest, state-of-the-art medical screening and treatments from now on.

When you get your bill for services that aren't covered by your insurance:

▶ **Don't complain. We're taking action.**

▶ **Get out your checkbook.**

▶ **Write a check to the healthcare provider, laboratory, or imaging company on the bill for an amount equal to that listed in the "amount due" section.**

▶ **Repeat this process as needed.**

▶ **Please never ask me or any other doctor to commit fraud.**

Nothing against the patients I quoted. We worked it out and I'm still their doctor. But since when did Americans stop being responsible for their health and well-being? How did the idea of buying insurance to cover an unexpected illness or injury become something that is expected to pay for every kind of preventive screening, every elective procedure, and every medication, including birth control pills and Viagra?

This all-encompassing expectation is unique to healthcare. We expect nothing of the sort from any other insurance we buy. Think about it.

Car insurance will pay to repair our vehicles after an accident, but we don't fly into a rage because it doesn't cover oil changes, new tires, new brakes, or routine engine repairs. Of course, if this maintenance is not performed, the car will either crash or break down, perhaps frying its engine or transmission, never to run again. So we pay to have it done.

Homeowners insurance will cover fire, theft, or plumbing damage, but we would never expect it to reimburse us for replacing a leaky roof, unclogging stopped-up pipes, or maintaining the lawn. Homeowners do these in their own best interests, to protect their biggest and most valuable material possession.

What *would* happen if our home and car policies started to assume these additional responsibilities for maintenance and check-ups? The public would expect all types of enhancement services and upgrades to be covered. Imagine what it would cost to buy insurance that would pay whenever someone wanted to replace carpet with wooden floors or get a custom paint job on their SUV?

Comprehensive "car-care" policies would be so expensive that many would drive without insurance. That would be a bad thing. Consumers would beg to go back to a time when home and car maintenance was their own responsibility, but insurance for accidents and natural catastrophes was affordable.

Yet the bizarre expectation of "total coverage" is exactly how people feel about healthcare. We pay an insurance premium, either on our own, as taxes, or as a part of our compensation for working, and we expect it to cover just about everything related to healthcare. I've had patients express outrage that their health plan won't pay for them to go to a chiropractor or a massage therapist, or if they do, only for a limited number of visits.

If I could have a free massage or a chiropractic adjustment whenever I felt like it, I'd probably make daily appointments.

If the public demands coverage for birth control pills, companies compete with each other to provide coverage for birth control pills, and the only way they can do that is to increase their fees to everyone, not just those who use the pills. When healthcare systems provide vaccinations for our children, that cost is passed on—not only the cost of the vaccination, but all the associated paperwork and bureaucracy. Don't get me wrong. I strongly endorse subsidies to vaccinate children who are obviously at the mercy of society for preventive healthcare. But the cost rises every time we demand another preventive service or another new treatment from our health insurance.

The combination of health insurance and Social Security has cost us a lot through the years, and it's only natural that we expect to get our value back. The result is the expectation that the system should pay for *all* of our healthcare needs. And that *expectation*, not the industry itself, is killing thousands every year.

Who doesn't enjoy bashing the government or managed care entities for their inefficiencies and bureaucratic stupidity. Yet we are willing to trust these organizations with our lives? Yes, many insurance companies are the model of a profitable, high-tech business, and not as inefficient as federal or state bureaucracies. And they make a lot of money for their investors, so they must be doing something right. But profitable or not, they serve what may be one of the most inefficient, poorly-run bureaucracies on the planet: the vast network that makes up the healthcare delivery system.

How can a financial entity, a thing that exists primarily to make a profit or to manage tax dollars, make the quality of our healthcare their top priority? When did we let them become part of our daily lives at all?

How would you feel if your car insurance company started telling you which gas you must buy and when you could and couldn't buy it, which mechanics you could use and whether or not you deserved roadside service?

By giving the health insurance industry responsibility for *routine* healthcare, we gave them the power to determine what is and isn't "medically necessary," which doctors they will pay for, how often we should get a checkup, a screening lab test or an X-ray, and which medicines doctors are "allowed" to prescribe.

Many of us have gone a step further. We now accept that we *can't have* a recommended test, purchase a superior medication, or see the doctor of our choice because it isn't covered by insurance. It is amazing and unnerving that people let some invisible third party determine the content and scope of their healthcare.

This passive attitude conjures up the disturbing image of a mindless herd of cows being driven from one pasture to another and eventually to the slaughterhouse. There may not even be anything *physically* keeping each cow from walking away from the herd except for the assumption that it can't. And when it comes to getting preventive healthcare, leaving the herd may be exactly what we should do.

There are no villains, no greedy insurance companies, or corrupt politicians to blame here. It's simply an impossible situation. Even if the insurance industry and the government healthcare programs weren't bloated, inefficient, and wasteful bureaucracies, they would still have to deal with reality and the limitations it imposes. They can't provide all things to all patients with a *finite* amount of money.

I believe we doctors and patients must accept some blame. Physicians allowed big business and politics into their practices, and patients believe they are entitled to 100 percent coverage for everything.

It's great that many people have health insurance through their workplace or their taxes, but this delegation of responsibility to a "third party" encourages individuals to sign over ownership for their healthcare.

That is very dangerous. The more removed the individual gets from directly paying for their healthcare, the more healthcare seems to be paid with "funny money." Just as I don't *seem* to pay for the roads I use or for the public school my kids attend, healthcare, too, has become something for which we do not pony up our own cash.

The old notion that we pay the bill when we see a doctor just as we pay the barber, mechanic, and grocery clerk has been replaced with the expectation that some "Big Brother" will work out the money with the doctor behind the scenes, long after we've left the office. We may even feel cheated, indignant, or outraged if they don't. This contributes a great deal to the mess we are in.

On some level, I think we all know that it is not really our employer or government or private insurer who pays for our doctor visits, medical tests, surgeries, and medications. We pay the bill. The money our employer spends to cover our insurance premium is considered compensation—financial benefits we've earned but are not found in our paychecks.

We pay into Social Security/Medicare long before we ever see the benefits. That is actually a *fortune* in lost opportunity. In addition to income taxes, the government takes an extra 16 percent of every dollar you earn for these programs. If we could wisely invest that 16 percent from day one of our careers, it would be worth so much at retirement that we wouldn't need Medicare or Social Security to fall back on.

Of course *if* they had the option, most people would not invest that money from day one. I wouldn't have done so as a young adult. I wanted every penny I could get my hands on to *spend*.

Our government takes on the job of holding our money for us in order to help pay for our healthcare when we retire. We have a similar situation in the working population. It's true that if employers didn't buy healthcare for their workers, they could pay them enough extra in salary to allow each employee to buy insurance for themselves. But many employees who now receive health insurance through work *would not* choose to purchase it, even with a greater wage or salary.

Our attitude, that having health benefits should mean paying next to nothing personally for health-related services, has helped make sure we now pay more than ever to purchase those "benefits."

Sure, the marvels of modern technology and the latest genetically-engineered breakthrough drugs are expensive, but at least they add value to our health. Most people understand that a three million dollar Electron Beam CT scanner or a five-hundred million dollar research investment in a life-saving cancer treatment isn't going to be free.

Here's the sad part. A huge percentage of what we pay through employer benefit programs and taxes, supports an industry that contributes *absolutely nothing* to our health. The insurance industry, both private and government, is a famished beast that devours the largest share of healthcare costs.

It employs millions of people who push paper and administer benefits and are probably very nice folks. They are not, however, doctors, nurses, or other caregivers. The companies may employ a handful of nurses or pharmacists who are paid to identify legitimate reasons to decline a claim, but they are not there to enhance your access to care. They are not physical and respiratory therapists, X-Ray technicians, scientists, or medical researchers. They are middle men. And women. They work in a business designed to suck up every cent of your healthcare premiums and pay back the bare minimum for the treatment you receive.

Your money goes to pay the salaries, pensions, and benefits of those millions of employees, for offices, computers, state-of-the-art communication systems, advertising, legal and accounting services, reams of direct mail you receive and never read, and annual sales meetings on Maui. And they must also turn a profit to pay dividends to their investors.

On the physician side, I personally throw out reams of junk mail on a daily basis, generated by well-paid employees of these companies. They inform me, in grand style, of some new drug they actually *will* pay for, or they send me 20 pages of pie charts telling me how much more or less of *their* money I spend on this or that area of healthcare.

Maybe they assume I'll respond like a good "team player" and prescribe fewer and cheaper medications and services. How anything they do adds value to the patient's health I have yet to discover. They do not advance the science or application of medicine, technology, or education. They simply take credit for using your money to pay for some of your healthcare and pocket the surplus.

And how about this: For every person on *their* end who reviews my recommendation for a test, a medication, or a consultation with a specialist, I need to hire a person in *my* office to make that request in the first place. For each person they employ to finally pay me for seeing a patient, I must hire someone to submit billing, follow up, resubmit, and follow up again with the company. This is the required dance for weeks or months before they actually pay.

I suppose it's good for our national unemployment statistics that so many jobs have been created, but what does that contribute to your health?

Now add malpractice insurance to all the costs that do not enhance your health services. Another arm of the insurance beast provides "protection" against litigation.

Guess who pays for all these hard-working employees and malpractice premiums? You do, of course. It's no surprise that employers all over the country are hit every year with either higher group-insurance premiums or less medical care for the same price. It's all money they can't pay out in wages.

Allowing a third party to take on the fiscal responsibility of managing our healthcare has spawned a powerful bureaucracy, *The Healthcare Financing Industry*. When that happened, the original *purpose* for the industry—to pool funds from a lot of people to use on behalf of the unfortunate ones who got sick or hurt—became irrelevant.

The first and foremost priority of any bureaucracy is to ensure its own survival. And that takes a lot of money, which means for businesses and individuals, buying health insurance is very expensive. So is running a standard doctor's office. In my practice, we must hire over five employees for every physician, triple the need from about 20 years ago. The average family physician must see their first dozen patients each day, five days a week, just to pay the staff and office overhead. The doctor only gets paid from the patient visits after that, which means cramming more patients into the waiting room, spending less time with each patient, and leaving the office too drained to recall the passion that once brought him or her to the field of medicine.

When someone develops a serious illness like cancer or needs a triple bypass or delivers a pre-term baby, the actual costs are staggering. And they're worth it. This is what we need insurance for—the unexpected, catastrophic events.

Not prevention. It is neither unexpected nor catastrophic, and it doesn't cost a million dollars. It can be planned for and budgeted well in advance. We don't do it because we think of it as really expensive and not our responsibility.

It would be wise to change this thinking. Consider preventive healthcare as an "essential, affordable investment in living longer and healthier," one of those things no one is going to pay for except you—like your car, rent or mortgage, or shoes for the kids. Yes, you could survive in this country without paying for these things, but life would be harder, less fun and leave you at the mercy of others. Likewise, you must choose whether you want the state-of-the-art health screening and risk-reducing therapies aimed at ensuring you don't suffer an early death because of a missed opportunity. That's a stupid reason to die.

As you know, many basic health screens, such as mammograms, PAP smears, and prostate cancer screening *are* covered by most health plans. But new advancements in screening technology are not. When I started writing this book, a colonoscopy was not a covered test in most benefit plans. Today it is. After being available for how many years? This vital procedure searches for colon cancer when it's still in a stage that can be cured. For years, patients had to cough up about $1,500 for the procedure. Many patients actually signed up for the test only to back out when they learned their insurance would not pay them back. And that was too bad, because a lot of people would have survived colon cancer if it had been detected and treated in time.

Colonoscopy didn't *just recently* become the smart thing to do. We've known it's superiority over other, less expensive, tests for more than a decade. It just took ten years and a lot of deaths before the public and professional pressure succeeded in convincing insurance companies to stop calling it "experimental" and start including it in their benefit programs.

Mammograms weren't covered by insurance until the 1980s. It's painful to think of the many thousands of women who died because they didn't get one, just because it wasn't covered by insurance.

All advancements have to earn their place in the lineup of covered benefits, which is fine if the criteria for doing so is to demonstrate safety and effectiveness to the satisfaction of the FDA. In most cases, however, insurance companies do not rush to provide better screening or preventive medicine to their clients. The public must lobby for it, in the meantime paying for it out of pocket. Once it is in widespread use and the public pressure mounts, and sometimes after a few lawsuits, insurance companies agree to reimburse for it. Of course, the cost will then be passed onto you, me, employers, and hospitals.

If the cost of health screening is partly included in your benefits, it makes sense to use them. However, if *everyone* with insurance made full use of their screening tests and treatment benefits, the industry would need to increase their fees again. Their rates currently reflect the fact that most people *under*-utilize part of their healthcare coverage. Even so, my suggestion is to use your benefits. You won't break the bank if you "cash in" on what you're covered for.

But the balance of the costs for state-of-the-art preventive healthcare must come from you. I'm talking about the tests and treatments that we *know* help save lives but are not yet covered by insurance, just as mammograms and colonoscopy were not included in benefits for many years.

The Electron Beam CT scan (EBCT), for instance, (discussed in Part 2) is not yet covered by any insurance plan I know of. So what? It's already a smart thing to do. It saves lives by finding heart disease *before* a heart attack, buying us time to treat the problem. It is not a smart thing to wait a decade for your insurance plan to share the cost with you.

EBCT costs about $200 and only needs to be done once for most people. An ultrasound to check for aortic aneurysms costs about $225 and needs to be done, at most, every four years or so to be effective. So far, we've added about $66 per year to the healthcare costs of an average 40-year-old. Add in other non-covered services such as special cholesterol testing to determine how best to treat a lipid problem, urine cytology to better screen for bladder and kidney cancer, breast MRI for certain high-risk women, an easily swallowed pill-camera for easy detection of early esophageal cancer. The total cost is less than $500 per year.

You could spend twice that much on lattes. Not all, but most people *can* afford state-of-the-art prevention. Yet, I know there are people out there who will flatly refuse to have the tests anyway. They are expressing their anger that their insurance company won't cover them. That'll show Blue Cross, right? Until people treat their health as generously as they do their coffee habit, many lives will be lost from conditions that are preventable or treatable.

That is a stupid reason to die.

"It's one thing to opt out of using the best in preventive medicine; it's another when we don't know it exists. Let's face it, a choice isn't really a choice if you don't know you have it to make in the first place!"

Chapter 9

A Deadly Gap

State of the Art. I love that expression. It conjures up an image of discovery and the emotion of pride. It represents the present day emerging from a long *continuum of learning.* It means progress driven by a desire for excellence, innovation, raw curiosity, and the yearning to create. The *state of the art* means the best of the best today, this moment in time, and the expectation of even better just ahead.

Today's state of the art in automobiles, for example, is a safer, more comfortable and fuel-efficient vehicle than existed only a few years ago. For years, I bored my poor wife with nostalgic stories of the 1968 Cougar that defined my youth. On our 14th anniversary, there it was in the driveway. What a trip down memory lane to drive the same car my dad had let me take to high school football games and on my first dates!

The ride down memory lane lasted about two blocks. What a *lousy* ride it was. It was like driving an ocean liner. It did not steer well, did not take corners, and braking was a nightmare. It was in great shape for a car that was the state of the art in 1968. Compared to today, it was a dinosaur. My highly-efficient, well-built, and safer Nissan will also be obsolete in less than 10 years. It's the same in medicine, except that advancements in healthcare are occurring much faster than in the auto industry.

Another expression. The *Standard of Care.* I think of mediocrity, apathy, inertia, yesterday's news. It's a personal thing, but *my* definition of the standard of care in the practice of medicine is this: The least amount of care we can provide without getting sued. It's callous, but accurate.

Our legal system views the standard of care as that level of care and expertise considered average in a community. Until that *average* moves up, the quality of care need not budge.

The accepted definition for the standard of care in the medical world is *that standard that licensed physicians are held accountable for in their practice.* In fairness, it helps ensure the physicians don't fall behind the times, and that's a very good thing. But there's a wide gap between this minimum standard and the state of the art that is available, especially in preventive healthcare.

Remember the Vienna physician, Ignaz Semmelweis, who proved that the "new" procedure of hand washing with an antiseptic would dramatically reduce maternal mortality? The fact that women died from infection as a result of bad doctor hygiene wasn't the only tragedy. The unforgivable thing was that they continued to die long after we knew better. More than 25 years of death by stupidity. That is a perfect example of slipping through the gap between standard-of-care and state-of-the-art medicine.

The lucky ladies who happened to be treated by Dr. Semmelweis in the 1840s, received the state of the art in infection control for their day, giving them a fifty-fold better chance of surviving childbirth.

Sometimes we get a wrong idea in our head that makes matters worse, and once we learn the truth, it still takes years for a bad practice to end. In the 14th century, whipping oneself was considered a standard treatment for the Black Plague. The belief was that the disease was God's punishment for sinning. Divine forgiveness (and survival) required self-torture as a demonstration of repentance.

It's hard to know when healers recognized that this treatment was not so effective. Speaking out was heresy, punishable by death. So that gap lasted for centuries.

Today, the lag time is not as long, thanks to instant communication and a pleasant reduction in the fear-based slaughter of intellectuals and scientists in most of the world.

It's unlikely that we've overlooked too many fundamental discoveries as meaningful as the benefits of soap and water. But there are an incredible number of small medical breakthroughs emerging hundreds of times faster than a century ago, and many have not yet made it into the standard-of-care category.

Apply the state of the art for each new breakthrough, and the benefits begin to add up. Just as it paid to be on the cutting edge of hand washing in 1840, it pays to use the cutting edge of screening and prevention in 21st-century medicine.

How does progress really happen?

I think most of us would agree that advances in modern semi-invasive surgery, the latest monoclonal treatments for cancer, painless imaging that can find a tumor the size of a BB, and a 99.9 percent reduction in polio are all good things. Each is now part of the standard of care, but at one time didn't exist at all. How does medical progress happen? Is our government feverishly investing our tax dollars to push back the disease frontier? You know better. Except for a tiny drop in the bucket funded by the government, the enormous advancements in modern medicine are paid for by private industry.

Let's look at a similar phenomenon in the world of computers. A few decades ago, computers were huge, multimillion-dollar investments that only governments and corporate giants could afford. One computer took an entire room that had to be climate controlled. The handful of companies that purchased them raised the bar for what business could accomplish with the miracle of a mainframe.

In order to remain competitive, other companies followed suit, creating a fast-growing demand for business computers. Increased demand led to mass production, more hardware and software companies, and rapid advancements in computer technology. It also led to lower purchasing costs, which small businesses could then afford, and eventually to the life-altering development of personal computers.

You know the rest. The average American home now boasts more computing power than was available on the entire planet 50 years ago. For the price of a TV, individuals can now join a global community in accessing and transferring information. The small segment of wealthy corporations and individuals created the market that now allows the majority of Americans access to the most powerful communication tool in history. Some people resent the wealthy for getting the best things first, because they do not understand how that ultimately benefits them.

The Damn Pharmaceutical Companies

So it goes with the pharmaceutical industry. Aside from being accused of conspiring to push dangerous drugs into the market, they are charged with price gouging, perceived as valuing profits above human lives. The general pubic believes the drugs many people NEED have become luxuries only the rich can afford. Some want the government to take control, forcing drug companies to lower their prices.

I am not one of those people. If treatments currently on the market are critically needed now to prevent and treat disease, it's safe to assume we are going to NEED many of those now being developed deep in the pharmaceutical research facilities.

Finding and developing new medicines is one of the most financially risky businesses in the world. It is not easy to get investors to finance such huge risks. The only way you're going to get a rational human to take *that* leap of faith is to provide a *potential* payoff to match the risk. In other words, the pharmaceutical company stock must increase in value.

This is the engine that drives drug companies to invest hundreds of billions of research dollars, raised through private investment and from their profits, into the discovery and production of new medicine and technology. The competition is fierce, and it drives the industry to work frantically to find new cures and treatments. Why? Because the winner gets *well paid* and stays in business. And this is an industry we NEED to stay in business.

Today, the cost for a company to develop a new drug is between $450 and $700 million. This covers the initial discovery of a promising compound through basic research, safety and efficacy studies, large-scale clinical research, regulatory review, manufacturing and marketing. In 1962, this same cost was only $4 million dollars.

The costs include the capital investments and research to discover and explore many compounds which never reach the market because they turn out to not be as safe or effective as hoped for. Only ten out of ten thousand promising new chemical entities make the transition from research to clinical development. Then only *one* of those ten drugs makes it through rigorous human studies and regulatory review to actually reach the market. The sales of that one product must provide the funds to pay for the 9,999 dead ends and for continued discovery and development of new life-enhancing and life-saving drugs.

Some industries simply matter more than others. The cosmetics industry has given us *Obsession* by Calvin Klein and *Curious* by Britney Spears. Competition in the pharmaceutical industry gives us products like the hepatitis B vaccine that will eventually wipe this disease off the face of the planet.

The time it takes for a company to recoup the costs of developing a successful drug is limited by the length of the patent on that compound. They have a total of 19 years from the beginning of testing until the patent expires. This includes the ten to twelve years it's being developed, leaving approximately seven to nine years of patent protection once the drug is on the market. After that, other companies can sell a "me-too" generic product that usually costs very little to produce. And once that happens, the medications become available at a fraction of their original price.

We can complain "better late than never" about the new, reduced price, or we can see the bigger picture that NO ONE would ever have had the use of a medication but for the possibility of a profit for those who took the risk of creating it. Now it will exist forever at a very low price, instead of never existing at all.

When I started medical practice in 1986, the medication Lopressor cost about $56 for a one-month supply. Patients complained bitterly but it did, after all, keep them alive after their heart attack or bypass surgery. Today, the generic version of Lopressor, metoprolol, costs about $4.95 for a month's supply. Is anyone thanking the creators of this life-saving drug that now costs a fraction of the price for a bottle of Britney's perfume?

Tagamet arrived on the scene in 1977 to forever change the face of peptic ulcer disease, once the cause of tremendous pain, suffering, and sometimes death. It is no longer a prescription drug. I can buy it over the counter for about the same price as Tylenol or aspirin. I can name hundreds of similar products, none of which would exist if the government regulated the "evil drug empire" in setting the price of drugs.

One of the main gripes about drug company policy is wastefulness. I've heard dozens of my colleagues in the healthcare field say that money spent on advertising and marketing is wasteful overkill. This marketing includes an army of sales representatives, expensive full-page ads in medical journals, nonspecific television commercials that end with "talk to your doctor," customized sticky notepads for the doctor's office, and expensive symposiums and other educational programs sponsored by drug companies. For years, a pharmaceutical company paid for my patient-related MEDLINE searches, a service that allows me to research millions of medical articles.

Obviously, these companies can't sell a new drug if no one knows about it. They have to compete in a very crowded market where every pharmaceutical company is trying to get 10 seconds of a physician's attention. I can attest to the difficulty of that effort. And in a world where patients are more informed, more actively participating in decisions about their treatment, it's important to make them aware of new developments as well. Although I'm in the minority of my colleagues, I support consumer advertising for prescription drugs, because it serves to start discussions between doctors and patients that may never happen otherwise.

While competition contributes to costly advertising, promotion, and customer education, which raises prices, competition also *lowers* the overall price of a product by increasing the volume sold and forcing a company to market their product at prices lower than would be necessary if they were the only game in town.

I'm not saying these companies are angels or even altruistic. They're businesses. Are they above lobbying in Washington to promote their profits and squash their competition? Not at all. They're ruthless. *All* industries fight relentlessly to gain and maintain every possible competitive edge. But if ruthless business tactics should be outlawed, then drug companies will need to get in a long line, along with the oil, automotive, mega-farming, telecommunications, weapons, and yes, the *food supplement industries*, to have their hands slapped.

So when you hear politicians talk about price fixing for drugs, keep in mind that price fixing in any field has done nothing but kill competition and, thereby, stifle progress in that field.

Had price fixing been in place 30 years ago, many of our greatest medicines would not exist. If you disagree, try to find some designer drugs created in the former Soviet Union or Romania. In the meantime, I will stand by my claim that this is one small area in which the capitalist model works really well. We all benefit from the lightning-fast progress in medicine when companies compete to create true value.

Like the first computers, the wealthy and the well-insured make profits possible by using the new drugs, despite their cost. That money makes the next drug possible. And yes, just like the computer, the rich or the well-insured get new treatments first. And that sort of thing just infuriates some people, *because it just seems so unfair*. Life is.

Three *Deadly* Assumptions About Healthcare

I've already talked about two of three very dangerous assumptions that many people make about the healthcare system.

The first we saw in the last chapter: *the assumption that we should expect our insurance or government health plan to pay for all things medical.*

The second: *the health system will protect us from preventable forms of death, injury, and illness.* Many young mothers in 1840's Europe learned the error of this assumption the hard way.

And number three goes like this: *in the world of medical care, everyone can and should be treated the same.*

Now, lets talk about what's fair and possible. *Everybody* benefits from the medical miracles in a free-enterprise system. But what angers so many well-meaning humanitarian advocates, is that not everyone can benefit to the same extent at the same time. If that was mandated, progress in healthcare would screech to a halt.

Will Rogers, summing up one of his remarkable insights about human nature, once said, "Communism is like prohibition; it's a good idea but it won't work." The same is true for one-size-fits-all universal healthcare. People with more money and resources get better care, period. That's why they strive to make money or have influence in the first place. They also eat better food, have better homes, and enjoy more conveniences than others. Their ability to purchase the best makes the best available to everybody—eventually.

Our feelings about the different tiers of society don't change the facts. This is how life is, how it's always been, and how it will be for the foreseeable future. However, people who want today's *state-of-the-art* healthcare for prevention don't have to be rich; they simply need to make it a priority over other non-essentials. True, it's not as fun as a new plasma TV or a weekend in Vegas, but the choice is within the financial grasp of most Americans.

Of course, there are many in this country who live in poverty. We also hear about the 43 million-plus Americans who are uninsured. These are not the same thing. I work regularly with the uninsured at a local free clinic, many of whom are employed, earning well above the poverty line, but need help paying for the *ongoing treatment* of their medical problems. Their long-term medications are provided for free by the drug manufacturers themselves, and our local medical community steps up to the plate to make necessary treatments affordable for them.

I have also been able to convince many of these motivated patients to *purchase* state-of-the-art screening tests for themselves. The costs are not prohibitive for most of the uninsured. I'm not saying that every community has the resources to help the uninsured pay for illness, just that screening itself is a small part of the expense.

For the truly poor, I do not have an answer. Safety nets exist through the nation's emergency rooms to provide life-saving treatments in a crisis, but the state of the art in health screening is not a crisis. It's a choice.

In years to come, today's newest life-saving medical advances will be dirt cheap for all of humanity. Of course, the newer, cutting-edge advances of that future day will still be expensive. Today or tomorrow, those who choose can wait it out. Those who want to take advantage of the best immediately, will have to pay for the privilege.

How many people are lined up to do so today? Sadly, very few, even in the upper-income population. But not because of the cost.

Katie Couric's late husband, Jay Monahan, died from colon cancer at age 42. He might have had another 42 years or more if it had been diagnosed early. When preventable tragedy strikes the rich and famous, it reminds us that money and influence are not the main barrier between life and a premature death. Often loved ones translate their grief into a positive commitment for public awareness to prevent others from the same preventable tragedy. I encourage you to visit The Jay Monahan Center for Gastrointestinal Health at **www.monahancenter.org.**

However, for every celebrity death that makes the news and inspires a contribution for a new hospital wing, there are tens of thousands of average folks who die the same way, for the same reason—a missed opportunity. They just didn't have the screening test, often because they didn't know they should.

Did actor George C. Scott, who died of aortic rupture, get the standard of care? Did Jay Monahan? Most likely. Had they received the *state of the art* in care, would they still be with us? Maybe.

For the past 20 years, we've had the means for identifying and treating the conditions that killed them. Jay Monahan's cancer struck him earlier in life than usual, and if he had no family history of the disease he may still have slipped by a conscientious screening program. But I'll bet none of his close relatives will. They now *own* that family history of colon cancer and will get the early screening demanded by his tragedy.

Why doesn't everyone at least *know* about the options available for finding such problems when there is still time enough for successful treatment? It's one thing to opt out of using the best in preventative medicine; it's another when we don't know it exists. Let's face it, a choice isn't really a choice if you don't know you have it to make in the first place!

Why is it so hard for the average person to discover what's available to them in this age of information? The answer, in part, is once again: *the standard of care*. It's the level that most healthcare providers become comfortable with as they wait years, even decades, for state-of-the-art care to become the standard.

It's a safe place to hang out, and safety is a critical issue for physicians. As long as they don't go too far beyond the level of care their colleagues provide, and as long as they don't aggravate insurance providers, they remain less vulnerable to litigation.

Once they embrace state-of-the-art medicine, they can be accused of going outside the "standard," a practice aggressively discouraged by peers, medical associations, and third-party payers who are not eager to pay for exceptional testing or medications.

In defense of physicians and other health experts, there are very logical reasons for resisting aggressive, not-yet-standard screening and preventive care. They want scientific evidence that these tests are really necessary and cost-effective based on large scale studies. Until they have the data, they do not want patients receiving care beyond the norm. They also do not want to be accused of convincing the "worried well" to pay for something that could be challenged as unnecessary or excessive.

In Part 2, I'll give you the information you need to assess the value and necessity of specific state-of-the-art screening and preventive procedures. You can judge for yourself if they should be included in your plan of care.

For physicians, it is not a good thing to be accused of spending too much or recommending not-yet-standard-of-care tests or procedures. That's how you get on the radar of powerful organizations like Medicare and the insurance companies. That's how you get scrutinized by local independent physician associations (IPAs). They all have a major interest in the scope and content of physician practices, and they can make trouble if they think you are coloring outside the lines. An accusation of over-treatment is also of great interest to malpractice attorneys who might not currently have a medical incompetence case to occupy their time. So the safest place to practice medicine today is smack dab in the center of the standard of care for your community.

There's another reason you may not know about your options. Physicians often assume patients will not want anything that isn't covered by their benefit plan and will be upset at the suggestion.

Many people have cosmetic surgery for which they pay out of pocket. Physicians accept this and don't think twice about it. Yet I often hear physician colleagues say things like, "*I had to* switch her from Zocor to another medication, because her insurance no longer pays for Zocor." Or, "I'd like to use an ARB blood pressure medicine because of the low side-effects, but *I can't* because his insurance says he must try an ACE drug first."

I *had* to? I *can't*?

Insurance companies don't really dictate what a physician prescribes. They just choose what they will and won't pay for. The choice is up to the doctor and patient. But whenever physicians assume they must comply with what is covered and what isn't, they effectively allow insurance companies to practice cut-rate medicine without a license. They may also fail to explain to patients why a non-covered treatment is better than one that is, thus denying the patient an opportunity to participate in the decision.

Another reason physicians don't infuse their practices with state-of-the-art care, is the considerable time it takes to stay current on innovations in preventive health. Obtaining current information about standard-of-care issues, on the other hand, takes little effort at all. Hospital bulletins, medical organizations, malpractice carriers, and pharmaceutical companies all help keep us updated as a matter of course. They each have a vested interest in doing so.

It takes a personal desire, commitment, and precious additional time to follow progress. This is in no way a put-down of physicians, many of whom struggle to see everyone in the waiting room during a 12-hour day that also includes completing charts and insurance forms and returning phone calls. Along with a chronically-overcrowded schedule, a bloated bureaucracy rules each day in the life of a doctor's practice.

The *latest* government mandate (check out www.hippa.org) requires all doctors, pharmacies, and hospitals to spend your dollars and their time making sure no one overhears anything personal about you. That's why you must stand 30 feet away from the pharmacist with cotton in your ears until it's your turn for service and why medical offices are decorated with placards warning you that *Auditory Privacy Is Not Guaranteed In This Area.*

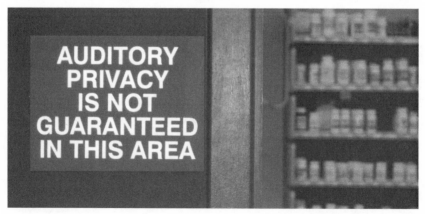

And oh by the way, to be even more compliant with this legislation, others must not *see* anything personal about you either, so in addition to the cotton in your ears, you may soon need to slip a blindfold over your eyes.

You must also sign a form letting the guardians of privacy know that *you know* your physician is complying with the law. Everyone in the health industry must also attend special classes to educate them on these vital matters.

Consulting services will now come into your office and help you sort out the law to make sure you don't get fined or jailed for being "non-compliant." In other words, we've spawned a whole new industry just to service this new law. And all of this just cuts into the time and resources available to actually help patients with their health. The vast majority of my patients just roll their eyes at the waste of time, money, and paper.

Clearly, our healthcare system has more important things to do than to spend precious resources informing us of our many options for health screening and treatment. There are, after all, important forms that must be filled out. So even though effective prevention is a subject that's easy to understand and can be made readily available to those who seek it, the people to whom we would naturally turn to obtain it are buried in the bureaucratic mindset of "what everyone else is doing" and what is "allowed." It just doesn't occur to most of us physicians to offer these options to our patients.

Did I mention our healthcare system is truly in a state of crisis?

It took a major change in the business model of my own practice before I was able to get my head above water to discover how much slipped through the cracks in caring for the three thousand people who called me "their doc." Like the majority of medical practices in the country, it was organized chaos day in, day out.

It seemed we were playing Russian Roulette with patient health. They usually had to wait at least 2 weeks to get a 10-minute appointment.

The devil lurks in the details of myriad signs, symptoms, and nuances behind the scenes of any patient's medical problems. It is simply impossible to uncover these in the required ten minutes. When it came to discussing and providing preventive care, I rarely had the luxury. It was all about the immediate problem, the one they waited for weeks to talk about.

Today, only 200 people call me "their doc." I know each and every one on a personal level. I no longer run into a patient at Home Depot embarrassed that I can't remember her name or whether she's dealing with menopause or breast cancer.

I spend an hour or more with each patient who wants that time. I can explain conditions and treatment in detail, advise them of state-of-the-art innovations they might consider and answer their questions. I can do this sitting down instead of with one foot out the door. I can *listen* to their questions.

I feel a huge difference in the quality of service I now provide, and the feeling is good. Likewise, most of my patients didn't really know how superficial their care had been until they started having all the details of their conditions addressed.

Return of the Small Town Doc?

The story of re-creating my medical practice ties directly into the gap between the standard of care and state-of-the-art healthcare. I now have a membership practice. Patients pay an average monthly fee of $85, which is like a retainer. It ensures patients access to my care when they need it, as often as they need it. I make house calls at no extra charge. Patients have all my phone and pager numbers and are guaranteed same-day appointments when they need one.

This means I get to deliver care exactly as I envisioned when I was in medical school. It means patients get care from a physician who knows them at a deeper level than what's in their charts. I no longer feel like I work in a quickie-lube type of practice as I now care for an *optimal* rather than a *maximal* number of patients.

And I collect a fabulous bonus—time. I actually have some left over every day. Time was once a luxury I couldn't afford. Now I can enjoy my marriage, participate more in my children's lives, write, lecture, and donate my services at the free clinic.

Some would call this an innovative way to practice, but it's really the way physicians cared for patients in the horse and buggy days. I just have the benefit of a century worth of advancements and state-of-the-art technology to go with it. There is a collaborative relationship between patient, nurse, and myself, and no more unpleasant or adversarial exchanges between an anxious patient and an over-worked staff. My support staff has the time to contribute to the patient's experience, which makes for a very positive, therapeutic environment.

Right now, however, practices like mine are controversial. Detractors claim that they are only for the wealthy and are unfair because they set up a two-tiered system, one for the rich and one for the poor. I've been called "immoral" and "elitist," and some politicians would like to outlaw practices like mine. Some say it will further worsen the growing shortage of general-practice physicians as more and more leave their high volume practices to care for fewer patients. It's a complex subject and beyond the scope of this book to fully discuss, but my own experience with a retainer-based practice does not support the claims of those who oppose them.

My patients are a mixture of poor, middle-class and high-income. What they have in common is that they put a priority on personalized, state-of-the-art healthcare. They recognize that the membership fee can translate into lower costs overall. Conditions that need immediate treatment get treated immediately, not weeks later when they can finally get an appointment. And because I am more fully aware of patients' health status and conditions, I know when it makes sense to "wait and watch" or try a home remedy rather than race to the office.

Sometimes all they need is reassurance that a symptom doesn't require immediate attention, which saves them the cost of an office co-payment. I don't have to write "guinea pig" prescriptions that cost a fortune and then may have to be replaced with something else because of side-effects. I have time to let patients try samples provided by pharmaceutical companies and closely monitor the effects before writing a month's prescription. You'll recognize the value of that if you've ever flushed a $180 prescription because you couldn't tolerate the side-effects.

As for practices like mine leading to fewer physicians available to meet demand, I believe they will have the opposite affect. I was seriously ready to quit medicine altogether. It was draining my energy and providing very few rewards. Every day was defined by the pressure to see more patients to keep the clinic from losing money, confined by insurance and government employees making medical decisions, overwhelmed by paperwork and an unhappy, frustrated throng of patients.

For me, the answer was either to find a way to deliver care as it was meant to be delivered or quit. Every year, thousands of physicians close their practices, not to retire from old age but because they can no longer endure being puppets of this bureaucratic system. They didn't study medicine to become a commodity of the insurance industry or Medicare.

There *is* a doctor shortage in office practice, and it's getting critical. Medical students are rejecting the primary care fields—family practice, pediatrics, and internal medicine—in favor of more highly-specialized and lucrative areas such as cardiology, surgery, and anesthesia. Who can blame them? They can make five times the money for about the same level of aggravation. If I was just starting medical school, I'd probably do the same.

In the past, the lifestyle for a general practitioner was more relaxed and less stressful than in the highly-paid specialties. That was the tradeoff, a reasonable lifestyle for a lower salary. But the lifestyle has gone downhill, as has the salary. So we're losing from both ends as experienced primary care physicians close their doors, and fewer young physicians choose to take their place.

I believe that a rewarding practice like mine will attract the best and brightest *back* to general practice. Could patients afford them? The fact is, the extra cost is quite small and a bargain in terms of the quality of care it buys.

Yes, there are very expensive programs out there, costing up to $20,000 a year, and they are geared toward the wealthy. When the retainer fee is reasonable and affordable, it can be the best deal around.

Insurance costs rise steadily, 10, 20, 30 percent each year and *less* coverage is offered for all that money. But by paying a bit more *now*, patients experience a dramatic improvement in their access to healthcare. They have all the time they need with their doctor, and he or she has the time to be a true healthcare advocate on their behalf, not only on medical matters, but also for jumping through the hoops and over the obstacles that face the average patient as they navigate the passive-aggressive world of insurance.

There may actually come a time when insurance companies offer to send you to a retainer-based practice, passing on to the physician the increased premium costs. They will never stop competing for your business.

I hope primary care practice evolves towards this model, where a doctor has no more than a few hundred patients with whom he can establish a partnership focused on preventive health and effective management of illness and disease. It won't happen soon I'm afraid, and, until then, some people will get the benefit of progressive care before others do. And just as with the latest new drug or expensive technology, it will just anger the heck out of some people because *it just seems so unfair*. Life isn't fair, and I hope you won't wait for that to change.

In the process of acting in the best interests of you and your family, you will be helping accelerate progress that will result in a higher standard of care for everyone. We have the ability *now* to prevent death from infection, heart disease, cancer, and many other conditions. The catch is, they only work if we use them.

PART TWO

FIND IT. FIX IT.
(A SURVIVAL GUIDE)

"When you feel fine, why interrupt life to look for something bad? And when you're feeling lousy, you want the few minutes with the doctor spent getting you back to fine again, not looking for more trouble."

Chapter 10

Looking in All the Right Places

"**S**creening," probably the central concept of this book, can mean different things to different people. A "screen" in a dressing room is a barrier intended to conceal. In sports, the term refers to ways for blocking the path of the guy with the ball. Sun*screen*, sun *block*.

A screen door, on the other hand, acts as a filter. Air comes in; mosquitoes do not. A human resources employee screens applicants to identify those who meet job requirements. Miners search for gold using a sieve to collect rocks, eliminate water, and find their treasure.

In medicine, think of screening as the process of filtering, identifying, or eliminating health risks. We're not looking for treasure but for signs of trouble ahead, all easily disguised within even the most glowing, robust patients.

Too bad we don't have a version of airport screening devices that would allow patients to simply walk through an invisible detector that identifies every defective cell, damaged artery, and any other prelude to an early death.

Since the "whole body sieve" is not yet invented, physicians must check each organ, each body function, one at a time. Since a very limited number of diseases are responsible for the deaths of a tremendous number of people, imagine how much good can be accomplished by focusing our screening and treatments on these causes.

Health screening primarily focuses on two types of problems:

▶ **genetic traits or defects we're born with, and**
▶ **disorders or diseases that develop over the course of our lives.**

When someone is born with phenylketonuria, a genetic defect that requires a *very* strict diet to survive and grow, it requires only a *one-time screening* test to identify the problem. A person has the trait or they don't, so a single test tells all. Fortunately, every hospital in the country screens newborns for phenylketonuria within three days of birth.

The other type of screening is ongoing, meant to detect "intruders" that try to slip in unnoticed, and to stop them before they get away with murder.

Mammogram reports may show no signs of cancer for nine straight years; then, after a decade of screening, the results find a tiny cluster of abnormal cells. Three, five, nine, twelve years of normal results do not earn you a free pass to skip your annual mammogram. In cases like this, each screening test is like a single strand in a safety net, built to "sift" not only breast tissue, but *time* as well, to provide a year-by-year comparison of breast tissue structure. This disease attacks seemingly overnight, and within a year can be big enough to kill. Leave out a year and you have a wide gap in the net, through which a deadly tumor can slip.

For each type of screening, we must do so at a frequency consistent with the disease involved. In the case of breast cancer, that frequency is about once a year.

For colon cancer, it's more like every ten years, because this is a slow-growing cancer that only kills us if we ignore the search altogether. It's an insidious disease, easy to forget about when there's a decade between screenings. It's also a very treatable disease unless no one is watching for it.

Except for individuals with high risk factors, which I'll get to later, most people over age 50 should plan on having a colonoscopy every ten years. If everyone with no special risk factors did *just that*, colon cancer would be another disease off our list of leading causes of death.

Most of the screenings described in future chapters are like colonoscopy and mammogram: tests repeated on a regular schedule to catch various diseases. Once we find a potential problem, it's common to take screening to the next level and search further, often with the one-time-only genetic screens, to help us sort out *why* we have a problem in the first place.

If a person has advanced hardening of the arteries and high levels of blood triglycerides, a genetic analysis of something called their "ApoE genotype" might better explain why they are prone to this problem. This, in turn, would help determine the best treatments to lower their risk of heart attack. The results of this test matter, because different diets and medications are indicated based on specific test results.

Such "next level" testing and related information is often beyond the scope of this book and is best taken up from our website. Our goal here would be the screening to identify advanced hardening of the arteries in the first place. *Then* we would use additional genetic screening to help us design the best plan of care for stopping the disease process.

Screening works when it's done correctly and on a schedule that varies based on the potential disease. It's not rocket science. It interferes very little in your life or lifestyle, and it's a small price to pay for living better and longer.

Okay, just how much time do *you* have to set aside on your calendar? If you're a woman over 40, you're likely resigned to an annual mammogram and Pap Smear; and if you're a guy over 50, you're at least *aware* that your doc wants to goose you each year with the gloves and some K-Y jelly. Whether or not you submit to these indignities, this awareness is a good start. You may also know that screening for colon cancer finally made it onto the 'A' list for the standard of care.

Breast, cervical, prostate, and colon cancer are truly big-ticket killers, and even though most Americans don't come anywhere close to getting screened like they should, *knowing* about the screening recommendations is half the battle.

Now, how about this. Have you talked to your physician about when to screen for:
- ▶ **Aortic aneurysm?**
- ▶ **Kidney and bladder cancer?**
- ▶ **Coronary calcium burden?**
- ▶ **Ovarian cancer?**
- ▶ **Hazardous sleep apnea?**
- ▶ **Esophageal cancer?**
- ▶ **Genetic cholesterol abnormalities?**
- ▶ **Lung cancer?**
- ▶ **Testicular cancer?**
- ▶ **Malignant melanoma?**

And if not, why not?

We talked about many reasons why effective preventive healthcare is so uncommon. Economic, social, and "human nature" issues keep health screening well below the radar of most patients and some doctors. And, while a lack of caring on the part of our physicians is not a major issue, it would be disingenuous to ignore the fact that the "doctor's visit" experience itself can pose another barrier.

In today's world, everything is on fast forward: fast foods, instant photos, immediate online access to information, entertainment on-demand, speed dialing, instant messaging, just add water and stir.

Meanwhile, the typical doctor's office exists in the "land that time forgot." It can take weeks, even months to get a non-emergency appointment. Then there's taking time from work, finding a parking spot, and, of course, the mind-numbing wait. Usually, you don't leave in the same frame of mind as after, let's say, a one-hour massage. It's not convenient. It's not enjoyable. It's not drive-through.

So I imagine you primarily schedule a doctor appointment because you need to, because you're not well. When you feel fine, why interrupt life to look for something bad? And when you're feeling lousy, you want the few minutes with the doctor spent getting you back to fine again, not looking for more trouble—for things that *aren't* currently bothering you and that you probably *don't* have. After all, if it ain't broke, and you feel okay, why go looking for problems to complicate your busy life?

Which brings us to the final barrier, the reason why some healthcare providers oppose certain tests which I choose to promote: *There are some very real risks inherent in the screening process itself.*

As I might have mentioned, everything is a risk.

"In a world of instant gratification, we are accustomed to one-stop shopping and quick fixes. But we can't buy our way out of the fact that uncertainty is as much a part of living as risk."

Chapter 11

Health Screening: Consider the Risk

WARNING: Some very bright, well-informed and competent people in the healthcare industry will disagree with my opinions on who should and should not have specific tests for specific diseases, and why. I am not saying I'm right or they're wrong. It's not that simple. This is a murky area and physicians will approach these issues with different initial points of view and a wide variety of assumptions. These affect where individuals will land on a position.

This is a great opportunity for you to consider different views, find out where your doctor stands, and then decide what's in your own best interest, free of myth and media influences.

Welcome to Near Perfect World: Here in downtown Utopia, physicians serve tea as they take all the time needed to give you a complete understanding of all your screening options. Third-party payers are *delighted* to cover all of these tests – especially those that are state-of-the-art. But it's strange. People here still die for stupid reasons. How curious that so many decline the free opportunity to prolong their lives. Why the resistance?

Back here in the real world it's understandable that we'd prefer doing something, *anything,* other than reading one of last year's Readers Digests in a crowded clinic, waiting for some medical invasion of our body. Yet we all do plenty of unpleasant things on a daily basis. It's more than that.

For one thing, we create real emotional stress when we deliberately go looking for something we *do not* want to find. And that stress skyrockets if we actually *find* it. Worry, fear, and sleepless nights are harmful to our health, relationships, job performance, and overall quality of life. We'd much prefer to avoid stressful inquiries altogether, and most of us pull this off brilliantly with our procrastination and "busy-ness."

But the often-quoted "stress factor" of health screening depends on you, your attitude about getting ahead of health problems, and your ability to deal with any *uncertainty* uncovered by screening. We know how the general public reacts to an alarming news story on a health issue. Imagine the reaction to being told personally that a screening test for cancer reveals a potential problem. This happens often, even if the findings ultimately prove to be harmless.

To say medical testing methods are "imperfect" is an understatement. Sometimes they raise more questions than they answer. An abnormal result from a prostate-specific antigen (PSA) test, used to screen for prostate cancer, is not a definite sign of prostate cancer. It just indicates the need for further investigation. Such uncertainties, inherent in medical testing, form the basis for much disagreement in the medical world over various forms of screening.

In spite of the real-world imperfections with screening, I firmly believe the benefits of widespread use of state-of-the-art screening methods outweigh their shortcomings. Recall the power of thinking with the logic of a scientist and the savvy of a gambler who knows the odds? It's important to understand and compare the risks of *not* having a given test and to ask all those questions at the end of chapter 7.

Screening tests can be as easy as contributing a little blood and as un-easy as being probed in places that must give Mother Nature a good laugh. The screening available for one disease may be a lot better or a lot worse than that available for another.

Let's compare a screening colonoscopy with a PSA blood test. The results of the colonoscopy performed by an experienced, skilled physician, can tell with almost absolute certainty whether or not a patient has colon cancer. This cancer is on the inside lining of the colon, obvious enough to be discovered in plenty of time to cure it. The idea of a 6-foot hose inserted through the rear end is probably not your idea of a good time, although the procedure is usually painless. The upside is you can count on the crystal-clear results.

PSA testing is the simple donation of a little blood to screen for prostate cancer. It's now considered pretty standard for men over 50. But it cannot give us a simple yes / no answer about the presence of cancer. Plus, it completely misses prostate cancer in about 17 percent of cases.

Prostate-specific antigen is produced in excess by many prostate cancers but *also* by normal prostate gland tissue, especially when it's inflamed by infection. Historically, a value above 4 nanograms per milliliter was considered a reasonable, if somewhat arbitrary, dividing line for PSA levels. Anything above that level is considered abnormal. Research demonstrated that about one in four men with a PSA level above 4 ng/mL would turn out to have prostate cancer.

Don't get me wrong. PSA testing is a standard procedure in my practice. I'm glad we have it. But it's no colonoscopy. How we interpret the results is not simple and has changed over the years.

A family friend actually had cancer that I could have identified *before* his PSA got above 4 had I recognized the trend of his annual PSA results. His levels went from 1.4 to 3.1 over the course of a year, still in the normal range. When his PSA level was over 5 at follow-up exam number three, his cancer was diagnosed on the basis of a follow-up biopsy.

On the other hand, several of my current patients who *do not* have prostate cancer, walk around with PSA levels between 5 and 10. Others have high levels intermittently for reasons such as infection.

PSA testing is like a moving target with a lot of decoys. Why isn't there a screening exam as reliable as colonoscopy for detecting prostate cancer?

The prostate gland is solid and about the size of a large walnut. Cancer can start deep within the gland and grow very slowly. Our imaging tools are not yet refined enough to find these small, deeply-buried tumors. We get to them with a biopsy by sticking a needle into the gland to get a "core sample," an invasive and often painful process. It's not something every man with elevated PSA needs. We reserve it for patients with additional warning signs.

The ambiguity of the PSA test makes it a good example of the grey areas of screening. Bear with me in this second and final reference to statistics. It's easy, I promise! And it's important. I can sum it up in two words: *sensitivity* and *specificity.*

The concept of sensitivity is fairly straightforward. Will our test find every cancer? Let's say we want to test a new and, we hope, improved prostate screening procedure in a group of 1,000 men. Fifty of these men have already been diagnosed with prostate cancer and we know the remaining 950 do not have it. Hurray! Our new screening test identifies all 50 of the patients with prostate cancer. It is therefore highly sensitive, and that can be a really good thing. But wait, don't open the champagne yet.

The test results are actually positive for 525 of those in the study. A "positive" test result in the case of screening means the test found a problem. Our new screening method *does* identify all 50 patients with prostate cancer, but it also indicates cancer in 475 men we know do not have it. They have a *false*-positive test result which means our new weapon is too sensitive to be of much use. The average *healthy* person would have a 50/50 chance of being needlessly scared from a false-positive result.

A negative result, however, could be very reassuring since it appears that this overly sensitive test is very *unlikely* to miss an existing cancer. If it suggests you do not have cancer, you can take that knowledge to the bank.

Alas, the super-sensitivity of this test means it would not be a celebrated breakthrough. The goal is to be able to both find the problem when it exists and not imply it's there when it isn't. This takes us to *specificity*.

So let's look at another "new" PSA test. This one does not give any false-positive results for our 950 cancer-free men. Great, except that it only identifies 10 of the 50 existing cancers cases. This test is very specific in that it never scared anyone who didn't actually have cancer. Apparently, if it suggests you do have cancer, you better plan to take action. But it's hardly ever going to say that! Even when cancer is growing exponentially in an unsuspecting patient, this test will fail to notice it 80 percent of the time! Sadly, this highly specific test isn't nearly sensitive enough to be of any practical use.

In Utopia, screening tests have 100 percent sensitivity and 100 percent specificity. Unfortunately, there is no such thing back home in real life. Colonoscopy is much closer to the ideal than a PSA test, but it's the exception to the rule. That leaves us with compromises. With PSA testing, our goal *cannot be* to rely on a simple blood test to determine who does and who does not have prostate cancer. The good news is that we *can* use the results of PSA screening very effectively.

For example, part of screening for prostate cancer includes the annual physical examination of the prostate gland, a.k.a., the finger wave. This helps detect the few tumors that don't raise PSA values.

The prostate gland can be felt very directly with a rectal exam. We also use the most powerful medical tool in our bag of tricks: the written chart. We record subjective findings of the physical exam that can be compared to the previous year's exam and the ones that follow. We note any change, such as an increase in size, a hard spot, or a lack of symmetry to the gland that wasn't there before. Low tech. Highly effective.

Next, we use that medical record to track PSA results, watching for increased values over time. If there is an increase, it is not a reason for panic, because the prostate gland tends to get bigger with age which may cause a slow rise in PSA levels. The change simply prompts a closer look. Perhaps the test will be repeated in three months instead of waiting a year to see if there's an upward trend. Normal aging is not likely to increase PSA levels significantly in just three months.

Even with a big jump in the PSA level, it's still not time to panic, especially if a tumor isn't found during the physical exam. Before more extreme measures like a biopsy are indicated, the physician can try a simple course of antibiotics in case there's an underlying, undetected infection. After the course of treatment, the PSA test can be performed again to determine if levels have returned to normal, something that won't happen if cancer is the cause. There is also an additional blood test called "percent free PSA" that can help refine our screening, but we'll leave that for the chapter on Prostate Cancer.

The point is there are screening tests like PSA that are not sensitive and specific enough to set off alarms but are still important in the search for conditions that can be treated successfully.

If this year's test is normal, say a value of 2.1 but last year's was only 0.9, then the screen should be considered slightly abnormal. If closer watching reveals that it's trending up rapidly, we need to know why. But conversely, if this year's test is clearly abnormal, over a value of 4.0, that *does not* mean it's time to start cutting! Is it higher than last year's? Is the physical exam consistent with a tumor? Could the patient have prostatitis that would respond to antibiotics? Does the percent free PSA blood test suggest a higher chance of malignancy? Only when all these questions are answered should the next step be considered; in this case, a needle biopsy of the prostate gland.

But how would *you* feel and react to a positive PSA result from *your* blood? Say you've gone through life with no more than your wisdom teeth pulled or maybe a knee operation up until the age of 52, and suddenly your PSA jumps from 1.9 to 5.3 in one year. You now have a 25 percent chance of prostate cancer brewing in your innards. Do you want to sit around and wait for the problem to advance for several months while your doctor sits on his hands and looks for confirmation of a trend? Or do you want to take action, find it right now, and kill it if it's there? After all, you've got a wife, two kids still in school, and no grandchildren yet to spoil!

But it turns out that aggressive over-reaction to a test can be as harmful as not getting screened in the first place. We really do have time to think and play it smart. When found through PSA testing, prostate cancer is usually curable for quite some time. There's no need to panic and rush into unnecessary biopsies, which are definitely no picnic and can cause bleeding, infection, and, rarely, some chronic problems. Plus, it gives sensible screening a bad name when our imperfect tests are used as an excuse for premature, often needless action like an invasive biopsy. I have personally NEVER lost a patient to a prostate cancer that I found by screening; and I've found a lot of them.

A big problem with screening tests is the uncertainty they may generate. It's the pits. This is why some physicians are unhappy with PSA testing. They do not want patients to be alarmed unnecessarily. Some people, especially the elderly, really can become sick with worry.

On the flip side of "worried sick" are the forceful, "take charge" patients determined to hunt down and hack out any invader. They would usually fare much better to relax a bit and wait. The outcomes of prostate cancer screening turn out much better overall with thoughtful, ongoing *management* rather than with a first-strike attack.

Who wants to wait to find out if something bad actually exists by waiting for it to get worse? For the patient, it means living for a while with a potentially serious unknown. We like things fixed. *Now.* Close, ongoing medical surveillance can extend for years, and in my experience patients *hate* that, especially men.

Ongoing management is a far cry from the "fix and forget it" approach we'd all prefer. It requires communicating with the patient and paying close attention over the years. In other words, the person has to be "in the system," not always a comfortable place for patients or the physicians who must keep track of them.

This is where our culture and the Baby Boomer generation need to "get real." In a world of instant gratification, we are accustomed to one-stop shopping and quick fixes. But we can't buy our way out of the fact that uncertainty is as much a part of living as risk. Our pervasive expectation that problems must be solved immediately affects medical practice, pressuring reluctant physicians to take some actions before they are either necessary or wise.

Screening Danger # 1: The stress and fear of uncertainty

Uncertainty naturally creates stress and fear, whether it's waiting to hear if you got that job or if you "passed" your colonoscopy test.

It's the first of four very real dangers of any screening test. However, I know *with certainty* that stress and fear can be reduced for all but the most neurotic patient. It's simply a matter of involving patients in their plan of care.

Low-stress patients are those who understand the benefits and risks of screening, how it works, and what it reveals, exactly what the results will mean, what they *don't* mean, and the steps that can be taken based on the results. They know what kind of "safety net" will be in place if the news isn't great. It takes an investment of time between patient and physician to develop that understanding—*before* the test is performed. The pay-off is that they become partners in their plan of care, actively involved, instead of feeling like a pawn in a medical game of chess.

Screening Danger # 2: *Another* test

We've already seen how one screening test can indicate the need for another. Since we don't have simple, perfect tests, we must manage this reality.

Some extra testing is pretty harmless, like repeating an abnormal blood test. Others, like an x-ray scan, invasive procedures, taking biopsies, or inserting cameras and instruments where Mother Nature never intended, are worthy of caution. Radiation and sharp objects can hurt people. This is why we must not overreact to equivocal test findings.

Runaway testing can also work insidiously in a person's self-image, even creating a "professional patient." This is especially tricky with people who generally don't feel great in the first place and don't know why. They are looking for the reassurance of a label. This book is meant primarily for the readers who currently feel well, but I have patients with chronic fatigue or pain who would like every kind of test that exists to validate their suffering. Finding a "real" disease would even be a relief.

I learned that for every screening test I recommend for a patient to undertake, I should have a response in mind for whatever result we find. This is especially important in my case because I'm aggressive in preventive screening, meaning I may get more false-positive results than average in a typical medical practice. I must take this into consideration when going forward with my patients. Watchful waiting is often the correct response to an abnormal result, so patients need to be prepared for this *before* they undergo a test in the first place. On the other hand, if additional testing is clearly called for, there is no reason to hesitate.

Screening Danger # 3: Danger from the test itself

I often argue that we let a "scarcity mentality" drive us to rationing important medical measurements and screening tests. Computers check the fluid pressures and oxygen levels on the space shuttle every millisecond or so, because even a small change can be a sign of something catastrophic. Shouldn't we be willing to be just as thorough with monitoring our bodies?

If we were machines with replaceable parts, the answer would be yes. But if I were to draw blood from a person everyday to make sure that there was no evidence of anemia, by the end of a month our patient really would be anemic thanks to my screening enthusiasm.

Again, some tests are pretty harmless like *occasional* blood checks, ultrasound scans, and probably MRI scans that use strong magnets and weak radio waves. Aside from the possibility of a claustrophobia attack—common, or a flying steel object left too close to the machine before it was turned on—thankfully, *not* common, MRIs have demonstrated no direct danger from the forces used to peer inside us.

Testing that involves hard radiation or sharp objects must be considered in a different light. We stopped the routine use of chest x-rays decades ago because it was of little value in finding diseases such as lung cancer in time to stop impending death. It was also intuitive that the accumulated radiation exposure certainly wasn't helping anyone. Likewise, do enough biopsies, and you'll run into the occasional serious complication. "Biopsy" is just another name for a form of surgery.

Even a physical examination has some risk. I once performed a rectal exam on a healthy guy that caused him to develop thromboses, blood clots, of his hemorrhoid veins requiring surgery! I felt awful. He felt worse. This exam is performed millions of times each year, but we cannot forget that there is nothing natural about inserting a gloved finger, however gently, up a rear end.

Clearly, injury from our screenings and examinations, including those that use x-rays or scalpels, is very rare or we wouldn't even be allowed to do them. Since you're now a statistics expert, you can confirm that the risk of a modern *routine* screening test is negligible, especially compared with the risk of avoiding it. But as the stakes get higher, such as a nodule seen in the lung that keeps getting slightly larger with successive CT scans, the need to accept greater risk makes sense. A lung biopsy is no small thing, but the *risk* would be heavily outweighed by the *need* in such a case. We must weigh the benefits and risks of every test with every patient in every unique situation.

Screening Danger # 4: Breaking the bank

There are those who claim that widespread, universal health screening would break the bank of insurance companies, Medicare, and Medicaid. They're not far from wrong.

Much like Mother Nature, insurance companies and government programs aren't concerned about you, a one-of-a-kind individual. They work with medical specialty boards and conduct extensive cost/benefit analyses to determine how many "net lives" can be saved by the widespread use of a given screening test. They compare that to the amount of money that would be spent to perform the test. If the yield is low—if it would cost a lot of money to save just a few lives, even yours—such a program is not considered cost-effective. It will most likely not be included in the screening policy recommendations issued by these agencies.

The average medical doctor then accepts the wisdom of the experts' recommendations—experts perhaps in reading actuarial tables, not in the practice of medicine. Yet, because they may give bladder cancer screening the thumbs down, many physicians don't even think to recommend it to any patient.

There exists a particular government-sponsored entity, the U.S. Preventive Services Task Force (USPSTF), which creates independent panels of medical experts to evaluate the available evidence on most available screening tests. They are more conservative in their screening recommendation than I am, but they usually provide a reliable review of the latest information available for each type of screening under consideration. For more information a about the USPSTF, please see Appendix 1.

However, purely *medical* review is not the only basis of evaluation by third-party payers who are concerned first about economic and only then about the medical implications of offering a particular screening. This is where some of my colleagues may confuse financial reasoning with medical value as a basis for the decision *not* to suggest certain screening tests. There is a big difference between not being cost-effective, i.e., being expensive, and not being worthwhile.

Here's where I part company with many in my industry. I do not base medical recommendations on coverage by health benefit programs since I do not expect insurance companies to pay for many of the screening tests I recommend.

As I said before, if healthcare premiums had to cover payment for all preventive care on demand, it would break the healthcare financing system in a week. I'm inclined to categorize the cost of most screening tests under the heading of Discretionary Spending. Like going out to dinner or upgrading my CD player.

There's no argument that financing the cost of universal screening for a very rare disease is not cost-effective for an insurance company. If you are at risk for a rare disease, take the insurance company out of the equation. It will give the idea of *cost effectiveness* a whole new meaning.

If the biggest effect of a test is to give you peace of mind, it has been an effective and worthwhile investment. When I underwent my heart scan and found no hardening of the arteries, the return on my $400 investment was huge. It gave me, as the saying goes, a new lease on life. No amount of dinners in our favorite restaurant could have matched that feeling. Had the news been bad, the value to my life would have been even higher.

When people elect to spend their own cash to give themselves the best chance of a long healthy life, how could anyone argue that it isn't money well spent?

Finally, my last point here is not about danger. Just discomfort. When you decide to take an active role in your health and well-being by seeking state-of-the-art care, you will be on the leading edge of next-generation healthcare. Your friends, family, and co-workers may not be there with you yet. Some people relish being first on the innovation wave, but many are uncomfortable being in front of the crowd.

My advice: for once, be the first kid on your block, be on the cutting edge. Be healthy. Live longer.

~~~

The Same Small Gang of Bad Guys

So what's out there waiting to kill us? More accurately, the question is, "What's *in* here trying to kill *me*?"

There are thousands of diseases that can kill, but the vast majority are uncommon or, so far, untreatable. Actor Michael Landon died of pancreatic cancer, and George Harrison died of a brain tumor; both had conditions that were beyond the scope of modern medicine. These are not stupid reasons for dying.

It is foolish to die at the hands of a disease that can be detected early and treated successfully. Many big-ticket killers as well as some uncommon but obvious troublemakers make the list. Of course, that list keeps growing. Every year, we make headway against formerly incurable diseases. Perhaps pancreatic cancer and brain tumors will join the line up before too long.

Here's my current list of stupid (along with some almost, but not totally, stupid) ways to die before your time:

▶ **Colon Cancer:** "I don't want to spend a day cleaning out my intestines so a six-foot tube can be inserted from the bottom up. Besides, it's gross."

▶ **Malignant Melanoma:** "It's just a beauty mark..."

▶ **Heart Attack:** "I'm cutting back on eggs, thanks anyway."

▶ **Esophageal Cancer:** "Everybody gets heartburn, right?"

▶ **Cervical Cancer:** "PAP Smear every year, I'd almost rather die..."

▶ **Aortic Aneurysm:** "Never heard of it."

▶ **Lung Cancer:** "I've already quit five times. It isn't going to happen."

▶ **Breast Cancer:** "That mammogram thing hurts."

▶ **Prostate Cancer:** "I pee fine. Why bother with a test even my doctor hates to perform?"

▶ **Bladder Cancer:** "Hey, I gave a urine sample."

▶ **Heart-Lung Failure:** "Ok, my own snoring woke me up sometimes, but who knew..."

▶ **Complications resulting from a broken hip:** "Don't need that bone density test. Every time I see that doctor he's got something else he wants me to do."

When I ask an audience whether they worry more about cancer or heart attack, the majority always pick cancer. Yet, in the last 24 hours, 4,000 Americans suffered a heart attack. That adds up to more than 1.5 million heart attack victims over the past year—*not* including strokes. About 900,000 of these people will die.

Cancer will have killed a little more than half as many, about 540,000 people, during the same year.

One-third of heart attack victims have no clue in advance; they figure it out when they're in the ambulance. Another one-third won't be surprised at all; they'll be dead before they know what happened. Their hearts simply stop pumping.

Most of us don't need to be convinced cancer is scary, common, and possibly fatal. But heart disease is public enemy number one. And it is actually a very slow, sneaky disease. People can be dying from heart disease long before death or even discomfort arrives.

True, many people die suddenly, some even in their sleep, which seems much better than being in the hands of cancer. But many survive the first heart attack and have to live with whatever remains of their heart. That means a high risk for congestive heart failure as the heart fails to pump with the speed and power our body requires. We become less active, our health deteriorates, and death comes in the form of long, slow suffocation.

So that's where I want to begin: behind the scenes of heart attack and stroke. Hardening of the arteries is a process called atherosclerosis. It can lead to a massive heart attack or a crippling stroke. It can also be stopped in its tracks if identified in time.

Following the chapters about heart attack, aortic aneurysm, and atherosclerosis, I'll describe state-of-the-art breakthroughs in finding specific cancers *before* they turn deadly, and finish with a few non-cancerous, non-atherosclerotic killers.

~~~

"A heart attack is the last step in a very long series of predictable and often manageable events."

Chapter 12
Anatomy of a Heart Attack

What exactly is a heart attack? How do arteries "harden"? Considering it's our deadliest enemy, it's ironic so many of us don't understand the process at all. This is largely due to the explosion of knowledge occurring over the past decade. It's easy to be left behind.

I want you to have a better understanding of what happens in hardening of the arteries and the disaster of a heart attack. These expressions should actually *mean* something clear and concrete in your mind.

Let's begin with a brief look at normal circulation: The heart pumps oxygen-rich blood, fresh from the lungs, throughout the entire body by contracting its strong ventricular muscles. The journey starts with blood squeezed from the left ventricle, the most powerful chamber of the heart. It moves through a one-way valve into the body's main pipe, the aorta.

The blood in the aorta and its large branches are under high pressure, the source of the grisly sight of blood spurting in horror movies and emergency room TV shows. From here, it is distributed throughout the rest of the body to each organ by dedicated branches of the aorta called "arteries." Each artery branches again and again until becoming microscopic capillaries. Here, the cells of the body extract nourishment and oxygen from the blood, and the spent, oxygen-poor blood returns through low-pressure veins to the right ventricle of the heart. The right ventricle pumps the blood to the lungs for fresh oxygen, then it's back to the left ventricle for another trip around the body. An amazing process.

The heart is the only muscle of the body that works 24 hours a day, 7 days a week. If it pauses for even a minute, we die. Obviously, it needs a generous, uninterrupted supply of blood for nourishment.

Yet despite the fact that blood passes through our heart's chambers thousands of times a day as it cycles through the body, the heart itself cannot draw any nourishment from the blood at this point. Like all the other organs, the heart requires its own dedicated pipeline system. This includes the left and the right coronary arteries and their network of smaller arteries, capillaries and veins, which distribute the blood throughout the heart muscle, providing food and oxygen to fuel the "endless" beating of our hearts.

These coronary arteries are tough little vessels that branch off the aorta just as it is leaving the heart, the first branches off the main line. They travel over the surface of the heart, then branch and penetrate to reach every speck of heart tissue.

They may well be the hardest working arteries in the entire body; not only do they carry a large volume of blood under high pressure every moment of our lives, but the heart itself is constantly in motion,

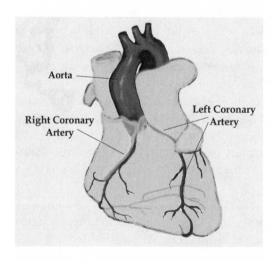

The body's hardest working vessels are the coronary arteries, providing the heart muscle with a constant supply of oxygen and nutrients. Now, we have the ability to know if something is interfering with their critical job.

stretching and contracting over and over. It must be a wild ride for the 70 to 80 years of the average person's life. The heart is the only organ that never gets a rest. Luckily, it has its priorities straight, which explains why the first organ it feeds through its endless pumping is itself.

If this blood supply is interrupted even briefly, any part of the heart deprived of food and oxygen starts to die. This is essentially what occurs with a heart attack, "gangrene of the heart tissue." You are probably familiar with the concept of gangrene of an arm or leg when muscle, bone, tendons, and ligaments die from loss of blood supply to the limb. The area eventually turns black and has to be surgically removed or falls off on its own. I know, it's a gruesome image, but it illustrates exactly what happens during a heart attack.

The medical term for the event is *myocardial infarction*, or MI, which comes from three Latin roots, *myo* for muscle, *cardio* for heart, and *infarct*, meaning killed.

An MI, a myocardial infarction, and a heart attack, mean the same thing: a piece of the heart has been killed. The person who lives through one does not heal from that heart attack, he or she just survives it. The dead part stays dead, and those who survive must live with the damage.

Fortunately, the heart exists in a sterile environment, so the dead tissue does not get infected in a way that requires amputation as would a limb. Instead, survivors develop scar tissue that replaces the dead tissue, and the remainder of the heart continues to beat. Occasionally, this area ruptures a few days after the heart attack, like a tire blowout. The result is death. Even when surviving the initial attack, if enough of the tissue is destroyed, the patient eventually dies from failure of the heart to adequately pump blood through his body. If the damage is less severe but happens to cause a "short" in the electrical circuits that trigger the heartbeat, the heart will beat so irregularly that it just quivers ineffectively; this is called ventricular fibrillation. The victim dies of sudden death for lack of synchronized beating.

Victims who survive without too much damage or a significant disruption in electrical activity get by with what's left of their heart. If the damage is minor, they can live well. If it's major, they may be unable to function at even a minimal level of activity without a suffocating shortness of breath. Most likely, continued survival will require many drugs to help compensate for the damage.

Okay, there's the grim look at destroyed heart muscle unable to perform its role of energetically pumping blood throughout our bodies. It's a bit like replacing a V8 engine in a truck with one from a lawn mower. Travel on life's highway becomes much more challenging.

What leads to this tragic event? What goes wrong to deprive the heart of its blood supply in the first place?

A heart attack occurs when an obstruction develops in a coronary artery, restricting the flow of blood needed to feed the muscle tissue downstream.

When this happens at the beginning of a coronary artery, the proximal end, it's like stopping the flow of nutrients in a tree at the base of the trunk. Considerable heart tissues dies, and the result is almost always fatal. When the obstruction occurs at the far end, the distal end, of a smaller artery, the area of damage is smaller and the chances of survival much greater.

The obstructions I'm referring to are not what you may think.

Many people think of "hardened arteries" as something like a drain clogged by gooey globs of fat that need to be roto-rootered clean. They may imagine a piece of this gunk breaking loose and traveling downstream until it gets trapped in a smaller pipe and plugs up the works. Or, they think the gunk just keeps building up until it closes the passage.

Nope. What actually happens is more interesting. It isn't gooey debris but the sudden formation of a blood clot, a thrombus, that abruptly stops normal blood flow. It's like what happens to prevent you from bleeding to death from a cut. In this case, however, clotting is not a good thing. The same process that stops blood from flowing out of the body from a wound, cuts off blood flow to a vital area inside the body in a heart attack.

Our blood chemistry means well. It's just trying to help, but the result is that tissue downstream from the clot dies from starvation without food and oxygen.

Why does this mistake happen and what does it have to do with cholesterol and hardened arteries? Is it just unavoidable bad luck, or is there more to it?

There's a great deal more to it. A heart attack is the last step in a very long series of *predictable* and often manageable events. Throughout our lives, a gradual process occurs called atherosclerosis. To understand it, we must first understand the structure of a hardened artery.

No, there is not a bunch of gunk stuck to the inner walls of our arteries trying to break free and float in the bloodstream. Nature is more subtle. Atherosclerotic goo occurs *within* the walls of arteries, not on the inner surface. If arteries were a rubber hose, fluid passing through the hose would not even touch it; the goo would be embedded in the rubber. There, it builds up over time.

In our analogy, this "rubber hose" is meant to carry a fluid that should not come into contact with this goo or even with the "rubber" itself. So the manufacturer added an ultra-thin, slick, inner layer, like a biological non-stick coating.

That's how our arteries are built, with a thin inner layer meant, in part, to make sure our blood does not touch the tissue beneath the layer.

This essential protective lining, the endothelium, is one of Mother N's most miraculous creations. A mosaic of flat cells completely covers the inner wall of every artery, presenting the slipperiest surface possible to enhance blood flow. It is amazingly thin, just one single cell thick, but does a masterful job of regulating blood flow and protecting us from evil blood clots.

If you enter a diseased coronary artery with a tiny flashlight, like walking through a storm drain, you'd see no change in the texture or integrity of the inner surface layer, even if there was a bunch of gunk, atherosclerosis, beneath the surface. You might find a slight inward bulge of the wall at the site, but the shiny texture would be intact, separating the blood flow from the gunk.

Life usually begins with healthy arteries, lined with the miracle endothelium to keep blood flowing and with no gunk on the other side. Over time, however, many of us build up complex plaques made of cholesterol-rich white blood cells that stick under the inner surface of our arteries. This is atherosclerosis. As long as blood never touches the plaque, life is great.

However, if the protective lining of the artery breaks down, peeling away like a bad paint job, the blood *does* touch the gunk which triggers the clotting process.

Blood, not having its own brain, doesn't know where it is in your body. It just senses when it touches something that doesn't belong there. Could be a knife blade. Could be a tiger's claw. Could be a rusty nail. All it knows is that something bad is happening, and it reacts exactly as it is meant to do. Blood platelets pile onto the area like the first infantry, determined to protect you. Along comes the second infantry with supplies including *anti*-platelet gear to make sure the first infantry stays in check.

But, if the plaque rupture uncovers a big enough area of the inner lining of the artery, the blood clot can grow big enough, fast enough, to bridge the entire diameter of the artery, creating a dam that stops all the blood flow. Unless the heart tissue downstream has a backup blood supply from other blood vessels, it's going to die.

If this happens in arm or leg muscles, it's not a big problem. An arm and leg can rest, take a break, which decreases its need for food and oxygen a thousand fold. The tissues affected by reduced blood flow can usually get what they need to at least *survive* from the run-off of other arteries.

Not the heart. It cannot rest. If it does, we die. It will plough through and exhaust any energy reserves it may have in a minute or so if the supply of fresh food and oxygen is cut off. So running out of blood for a few minutes is all it takes to kill heart muscle.

Many plaque ruptures and the blood clots they incite are too small to block the artery, and go away unnoticed. The area heals just like a scratch does: the clot covers the torn area to protect it while the endothelium grows back. The scab gradually dissolves, and life goes on.

The reason that aspirin in our system reduces the risk of heart attacks is because it slows down the pace of the platelets that pile on, thereby shifting the balance toward smaller clots that stop growing before they get big enough to block an artery.

There are also times, even with a complete blockage, that the heart tissue downstream is lucky enough to have an additional blood supply, small blood vessel connections to other arteries called collateral circulation, which is sufficient to keep it alive until the body can repair and re-open the vessel. The person may experience chest pain or shortness of breath when trying to exert him or herself, but at least the heart muscle survives. Unfortunately, for many people with a lot of atherosclerotic plaque, the rupture process occurs so often that eventually a thrombus blocks an unprotected artery.

So what's in a plaque to make it rupture? One word: inflammation. I doubt you share my fascination with this subject, but if so you'll find a more detailed discussion of the inflammatory process and related issues in Appendix 2.

In the process, these cells release substances that cause local swelling and other damage. This attracts more white cells which are always looking for a fight. When they sense damage in an area— even when it's caused by their own kind, they congregate. The crowd gets bigger and the plaque continues to build.

It can form in different ways, sometimes strong enough not to rupture, sometimes frail and vulnerable. Plaque that continues to grow without bursting begins to take up space, gradually narrowing the passageway of the artery over months or years without causing a catastrophic rupture and sudden loss of blood flow.

These large stable plaques probably account for some of the angina that many patients develop. They typically notice pain or other feelings of distress during exercise when their heart needs the most blood. Angina pain is from inadequate amounts of blood getting to part of the heart, but not to the point of killing tissue.

Because of the partial obstruction, the heart then outruns its available blood supply and starts to build up lactic acid, just like any of our other muscles do when we work them hard enough. Try holding one arm straight out to the side for five minutes, and you'll know what I mean!

Such symptoms warn people that something is wrong before some or all of their heart dies. Another amazing side-effect of this gradual narrowing is that the heart becomes aware of diminished blood flow and slowly develops or enlarges connections to other blood vessels to provide a small backup collateral blood supply to the endangered area.

Cardiologists love stable plaques. If you must have plaque, the stable variety is preferable. Ironically, people with the tough, thick plaques, who experience the warning signs of angina, are not as close to death as they believe.

Joe tells his doctor about chest pressure or pain up and down his arm. Doc goes ballistic and rushes him to the hospital. An angiogram clearly reveals a coronary artery more than 95 percent blocked. Either a stent is inserted to keep the affected area open, or Joe has open heart surgery to attach a new "hose" to the aorta and splice the other end to the coronary artery beyond the clogged area. Joe's blood supply to the tissue that was on the wrong side of the blockage is fully restored.

The return of robust blood flow feels tremendous and patients are often amazed to realize, in hindsight, how they had systematically curtailed their activities for months and even years leading up to the actual discovery of their clogged arteries. With immense relief and gratitude, Joe is convinced he was only 5 percent away from certain death—could have dropped dead at any minute!

Not necessarily true. He may have just been 5 percent away from feeling really rotten. Patients like Joe have often developed a backup blood supply, enough to keep the heart tissue alive if the artery completely closes off. In fact, it's highly likely that the original vessel actually closed off completely several times in the past only to be reopened again by the body's natural remodeling processes.

These patients feel terrible when they try to make their heart outrun the amount of blood available, and that usually stops them in their tracks. But at least they have backup to keep the blood-starved area alive.

I'm not saying that a person with angina never drops dead—even with a blood reserve from collateral circulation. Like Joe's doc, I would rush the patient to the hospital for an angiogram. But I want to distinguish between this situation and one that is more life-threatening and far more common: the patient with flat plaques that don't narrow their arteries significantly. Seems counter-intuitive, I admit, but give me a big bulky, yet relatively stable, plaque any day.

The flatter plaque is a prolific killer. When it ruptures and suddenly stops blood flow, it's a complete surprise to the poor heart that never saw it coming. Since the artery has not been narrowed, the heart muscle has never felt the metabolic stress from slightly outrunning its blood supply from time to time. Without this occasional shortage of oxygen, the heart doesn't get the warning it needs to create a backup plan of collateral circulation.

There's no safety net when a flat plaque ruptures and causes a blockage. That's the end of the line for the heart muscle that relies on the affected artery. This is why a heart attack is often the first sign that many people have of a problem in their coronary arteries. Whether they live or die will be a matter of sheer luck. One-third will die.

What's so very tragic is that up to a split second before the heart attack, the entire heart muscle is healthy, strong, and raring to go for many more years. Within an hour after its attacked, some of the muscle is gone forever.

It does not matter how extensive a person's atherosclerotic disease is, the heart itself is not damaged by the process until a rupture and the subsequent artery-clogging blood clot occur. Conversely, even with very little hardening of the arteries, when a small plaque ruptures in a bad place, the result is a major heart attack.

Millions of people in America, and billions worldwide, walk around with a lot of plaque in their coronary arteries. The good news is that modern medical treatments can stabilize plaque to prevent rupture and spare many of these folks a catastrophic heart attack. The catch is we have to know who these people are. That's the bad news.

Current programs for preventing heart disease *do not* focus on identifying those with cholesterol plaque. Think about that. Here is a glaring example of where the standard of care, even the standard of knowledge, is nowhere near the state of the art.

When we look for colon cancer, we take real-time images of the colon with a camera. When we look for breast cancer, we take real-time images of breast tissue. But when it comes to heart disease, we do not get real-time images inside the endothelium. Our screening, in fact, has nothing to do with viewing the circulatory system. We look at indirect evidence: the level of cholesterol in the blood, blood pressure, blood sugar, smoking, family history, and other factors.

These things matter, of course, but they put us in a dangerously ineffective paradigm that limits our efforts to prevent heart attacks. They are focused on lowering overall risk for a group, not for an individual. Like you, for instance.

"At this marvelous moment in time, it is possible to identify the causes of atherosclerosis in 90 percent of patients with hardening of the arteries. That percentage will get even better in the years ahead."

Chapter 13

Escaping The Big One

The risk for heart attack should scare us as much as the combined risk for cancer, AIDS and suicide bombers. Today's standard methods for preventing The Big One are sadly outdated for the 21st century. After all, our ability to detect and treat heart disease has come a very long way in a relatively short time.

For centuries, the best we could do was look for patterns that identified those who *seemed* more likely to suffer heart attack or stroke. A stroke is just a heart attack that occurs in brain tissue instead of the heart. To be fair, past observers, who did not have the advantage of current technology, made some very astute observations. They recognized the tendency for heart disease to run in families, and that people who carry their weight in their gut are at higher risk.

Obesity, elevated blood pressure, and diabetes were all correctly seen as undesirable traits in maintaining a healthy heart. In the 20th century, smoking joined the list, and as science and technology advanced, researchers discovered a strong correlation between heart attacks and high cholesterol.

In the 1940s, The Framingham Database was established to collect information on the test results, habits, and vital signs of *hundreds of thousands* of people living near Framingham, Massachusetts. The decades-long process of recording this information made it possible to create statistical models that accurately predict what percentage of a population is likely to have a heart attack or stroke within the next ten years.

Factor a person's age, gender, blood pressure, cholesterol, smoking status, family history, and a few other variables into the formula (Appendix 3), and it spits back a surprisingly accurate probability for an individual's risk of a heart attack within the next ten years.

If Jane's result from this assessment is 25 percent, it means she has a one in four chance of having a heart attack within ten years. That's bad. Such a high score means her information included risk factors like high cholesterol results and/or high blood pressure.

Her score would signal her doctor to focus on the specific problems that gave Jane such a high score. She can't change a strong family history if that contributed to her score. But high cholesterol or high blood pressure can be treated. If she's a smoker, maybe she will be motivated to quit.

So, that's the current method for determining who's at risk and what to do about it. Why is this a problem?

Because this approach is most handy for looking at risk in patient *populations*, and you are not a population. Doctors don't treat populations; they treat individuals, preferably one at a time.

Here's the thing: Jane's hypothetical score of 25 percent does not mean that she has half the coronary plaque of a person with a score of 50 percent or twice the amount of plaque as the guy with a score of 12.5 percent. In fact, Jane could have no plaque at all and live to be 100 with a perfect heart. Or, she could have a fatal heart attack the day she gets her score.

Her score of 25 percent simply means that if we isolated her with 99 other people who have the same score, 10 years later about 25 of these folks will have had a heart attack. Problem is, no one knows which ones.

So, physicians would treat everyone in the group. They would try to inflict restrictions on the diets and lifestyles of all 100, even though only 25 percent may need to change anything.

If, after treatment, only 10 percent actually had heart attacks, there would be no way of determining who actually benefited from treatment and who didn't need it to begin with.

Human beings are notoriously uncooperative when it comes to adhering to lifestyle changes or taking preventive medication, especially when the benefits are not absolutes and there is no concrete way for an individual person to measure success. And treating risk factors effectively means using medications, many of them expensive and not without possible side-effects. Theoretically, a physician could do more harm than good by exposing a patient to multiple medications if, in fact, they would never have had a heart attack anyway.

Until recently, if we wanted to prevent 25 lives from being cut short, we could only take this shotgun approach. We established a one-size-fits-all evaluation of risk factors, recommendations of lifestyle changes, and prescriptions for treatment.

If this was still the best approach we had, I wouldn't complain about it. But it's a new day, and we can do better.

We can check each individual *directly* for atherosclerotic disease of the coronary vessels. If we find it, we start the manhunt for the causes, and when we find them we prescribe *individualized* treatment to reduce the risk.

What if your friendly neighborhood heart doctor could put you to sleep, borrow your heart, and unscrew it to see exactly what's going on? What if he could hold your arteries up to the light to find and measure atherosclerosis?

You'd wake up knowing exactly where you stood in terms of heart disease. No significant sign of disease, and you go home happy. Some atherosclerosis, and you go home with a custom-made treatment plan.

If we were to put our 100 patients with the 25 percent chance of a heart attack within 10 years through such a test, what might we expect to find?

We would probably see that about one-third of them have no evidence of significant atherosclerotic disease at all. We'd be able to say with certainty that the odds of any of these 33 folks having a heart attack in the next 10 years are not 25 percent but less than 1 or 2. They'd leave the office with big smiles on their faces.

The other 67 would probably show some evidence of atherosclerotic disease, and a few more details could help us delineate them even further. For example, the health of a 75-year-old man who had a small amount of atherosclerosis, who quit smoking at the age of 50 and has no other obvious problems to account for his heart disease, would concern us less than the 42-year-old woman with extensive atherosclerosis. This is because, for the most part, atherosclerosis is cumulative.

So while it would be unlikely that our 75-year-old truly has the 25 percent chance of a heart attack that his Framingham score predicts, it is even more unlikely that our 42-year-old gal with extensive atherosclerosis will get through the next decade without major heart problems. Would we want to treat both people? Yes, but we would tailor our treatments for their individual circumstances.

Consider a 70-year-old woman with no evidence of atherosclerosis but a dangerously high cholesterol level. The conventional approach would compel us to treat her anyway, because we don't know for a fact her heart and arteries are fine. Her treatment would be based on knowing that elevated cholesterol is associated with risk for heart attack in a large group of people.

Today, knowing this woman has lived her 70 years without developing atherosclerosis, she can almost certainly be spared medical treatment for her elevated cholesterol. Whatever is going on in her body, high cholesterol is not hurting her.

Instead of making treatment decisions based only on what occurs in a population, we can now shift to really *assessing each patient as an individual.* We can directly evaluate what is happening in his or her coronary arteries. And we don't have to remove your heart and arteries to get this information. Knowing atherosclerosis starts many years before a heart attack occurs, we can identify *your* risk—now.

The number of known indicators for risk of heart disease has grown well beyond just high blood pressure, cholesterol levels, diabetes, family history, and smoking. The old approach of "look for all possible risk factors and treat each one," becomes impractical. To evaluate every person for each known risk factor would require thousands of dollars of tests, including things like C-reactive protein, homocysteine, lipoprotein [a], fibrinogen, plasminogen activator inhibitor-1, abdominal circumference, small dense highly oxidized LDL subsets, chlamydia antibodies, Interleukin 6, myeloperoxidase levels, and more.

A lot of testing, a lot of money, a lot of uncertainty, and a lot of wild goose chasing in the form of treatments that may not even be necessary. It means a greater burden on an already fragile healthcare system.

When we *concentrate* the hunt for new or obscure risk factors by focusing our treatments on people we know have an atherosclerosis problem, everybody wins.

At this marvelous moment in time, it is possible to identify the causes of atherosclerosis in 90 percent of patients with hardening of the arteries. That percentage will get even better in the years ahead. And the really good news is that we have extremely effective treatments that will benefit nearly all of them.

We need to get a direct look at each individual heart without putting patients to sleep and removing organs. The ability to painlessly do this is here now with an Ultra Fast CAT scan. These amazing machines are fast enough to take a picture of the ever-beating heart with such incredible clarity; we can actually see atherosclerosis lurking in coronary arteries. It is the most accurate way, to date, for identifying who's who in the search for future heart attack victims.

The alarming fact is that we've had this imaging technology for over 20 years and are only just beginning to utilize it on any sort of widespread scale.

"While waiting for the heart scan to be inducted into the standard-of-care hall of fame, while waiting for doctors to catch up with this technology, while waiting for patients to invest a few bucks in their own survival, heart attacks will continue claiming our loved ones long before their time"

Chapter 14

Know What is in Your Heart

Until recently, we would most often confirm a person had atherosclerosis of the coronary arteries *after* they had a heart attack or reported symptoms of angina. However, identifying a problem after half the heart is dead or during an autopsy is clearly not the goal of medical practice.

A person's electrocardiogram (ECG) pattern changes after part of the heart dies. Each person has his or her own ECG "fingerprint," and certain changes in the pattern allow us to confirm when they have already had at least one myocardial infarction.

A stress exercise test can help reveal a heart that outruns its available blood supply during exercise when the cause is a *partially* blocked coronary artery. If the heart needs more blood than it's getting, we see temporary changes in the ECG. We can also find and photograph partially clogged arteries with an angiogram, an invasive procedure.

However, stress testing and angiogram only reveal the effects of *narrowed* arteries, telling us nothing about the common, relatively flat plaques in our artery walls that don't limit blood flow at all, that haven't yet caused heart damage.

Yet these can be the most dangerous plaques of all, able to kill without warning at any time, because they are often unstable, inclined to rupture easily and cause a sudden blockage. We could run on the treadmill for hours or have a perfectly normal angiogram only to die five minutes later when one insidious plaque chooses to rupture.

The ultra-fast CT scanner provides a direct look at the coronary artery walls and can see cholesterol plaque, whether it's flat or bulky.

This scan predicts, *up to 100 times better than any other single risk factor*, who is in danger of a heart attack and who is not. This device solved the longstanding problem of trying to get a clear image of a heart that refuses to stand still to have its picture taken. Until recently, conventional CT scans required a full second or so to get each image or "slice." The result was a blurry, vague look at a throbbing heart.

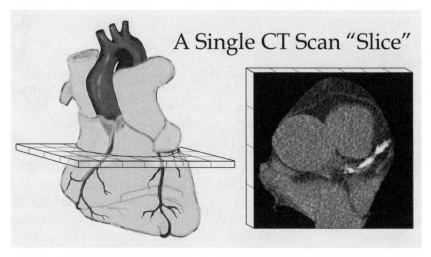

The Ultra Fast CT scanner creates a series of images of individual sections of the heart. It's looks at the heart in approximately thirty slices that give physicians the clearest, most comprehensive look at what's working right – and what isn't.

To speed things up, designers replaced the original moving x-ray generator and camera of a CT scanner, which rotates around the patient inside a big doughnut-shaped ring, with a high-energy electron gun aimed at a large tungsten ring surrounding the patient. The Electron Beam Computed Tomography scanner (EBCT) was born.

It is designed a bit like the TV picture tube in your home, which magnetically sweeps a focused beam of electrons across the screen many times per second, causing the screen to radiate the moving light and color that our eyes interpret as Sesame Street or a CSI episode.

But instead of radiating light, this electron beam causes the tungsten ring to radiate x-rays. And at lightning speed—because like a TV picture tube, there are no moving mechanical parts. The result is a CT scan image taken in a fraction of a second, capable of providing a clear image of the heart between beats.

Using this equipment in the late 1970s, researchers noticed some hearts had calcium buildup in the coronary arteries; others did not. But our understanding of heart disease then was limited. The potential value of this new ability to detect calcium buildup was mostly disregarded, except by a few mavericks who pursued research studies.

They learned that the more calcium seen in the heart vessels, the more atherosclerotic plaque existed. Some plaques contain no calcium and are therefore invisible to this scan, but a person with *significant* amounts of atherosclerosis has enough calcified plaque to be noticed virtually all the time.

It turns out that a person with twice the coronary calcium seen as his friend probably has about twice the plaque burden as well. If a person has no observable calcium in his arteries, long-term studies demonstrate that the total plaque load is so small that he's very unlikely to have a heart attack in the next five or ten years, *even if other risk factors*—cholesterol, blood pressure, family history—say otherwise.

This technology has been tested on over 40,000 individuals over the past two decades to determine how well it predicts future events and in the past few years, it has been the subject of many scientific publications. The technology works. The ability of high-speed CT scanning to measure the amount of coronary plaque provides a far more accurate prediction of a heart attack than measuring cholesterol.

Small wonder. It identifies the specific amount of atherosclerosis in an individual rather than identifying risk in a population.

In my practice, we have found a surprising amount of coronary artery disease in people who did not expect to have it, who didn't fit the traditional profile. And on occasion, we have been delightfully surprised by the absence of disease in patients we thought were prime for a heart attack.

The test requires less than ten minutes; you don't even take off your shirt. You lie on the CT scan table while two or three electrodes are stuck to your tummy. These instruct the machine when to take the pictures between heart beats. Take a deep breath. Hold. That's it. You're done. The images are often available immediately and sent with a written interpretive report to patient and physician.

The medical response to heart disease found by a heart scan is complex and changing. Quite honestly, many patients don't get the treatment they need even after the scan detects a problem. Remember our battle with the standard of care? If disease is there, we should expand our search for treatable, sometimes uncommon causes. More on this later.

Conversely, if a person has high cholesterol or some other issue, such as an abnormal fibrinogen or C-reactive protein, two newer and poorly-understood risk factors, a negative heart scan is cause for celebration. In addition to gaining peace of mind, the patient might be spared unnecessary treatment.

The established practice of identifying indirect risk factors for heart disease, such as high cholesterol, high blood pressure, diabetes, smoking, and family history is still important. When integrated with the results of a heart scan and individualized testing for related risk factors, we wield a powerful tool for providing treatment that is customized for the specific needs of each individual.

Today, conventional CT scanners, complete with their moving parts, have caught up in speed with the more expensive electron-beam type, which means more scanners are available nationwide and the cost is steadily coming down. Currently, the cost is about $200 compared to $400 a couple of years ago. That's a good thing, since very few benefit programs pay for this state-of-the-art screening test. If this lack of insurance coverage upsets you, please read Chapter 8 again to recall why leaving insurance out of the picture may be a good thing.

Here's what I would do next: *get the test.* If I didn't have an extra $200 on hand, I'd start saving. Because if it finds a problem, there are a lot of safe, easy, and effective ways to halt hardening of the arteries and to stabilize existing plaques to avoid a heart attack down the road.

Some experts recommend a scan for all men over 40 and women over 50 *if* they have at least one other "traditional" risk factor. I encourage my patients in these age groups to have a scan even if they do not have a single risk factor. I've found the highest (worst) plaque score in my friend, Frank, a 66-year-old man who never smoked and whose cholesterol, blood pressure, blood sugar, and homocysteine were normal. So was his exercise treadmill test. Without the scan, nobody would have considered him a candidate for hardening of the arteries.

The experts would not have recommended a scan since he had no apparent risk factors. In the subsequent search to find obscure risk factors, we found two that could explain the problem, both now being effectively treated.

I'll continue to follow his heart disease over the coming years to be sure the treatments are effective and to watch for newly discovered risk factors that may contribute to his problem. The bottom line is that if my friend did not have the scan, he would most likely have been on the road to a heart attack.

Of the hundreds of my patients who have had the scan, not one has regretted it. Whether they experienced relief at a negative test or had to face the fact that their arteries needed help, they were grateful to know either way. All agree it's better to be getting treatment for preventing a heart attack instead of struggling to recover from one.

There's no question this scan saves lives. Yet, despite the fact that it's been around for 20 years and research supports its value, it is not the standard of care. You will have to ask for it. Or, you can wait another decade or two, until physicians, insurers, and the general public no longer consider it new or experimental.

While waiting for the heart scan to be inducted into the standard-of-care hall of fame, while waiting for doctors to catch up with this technology, while waiting for patients to invest a few bucks in their own survival, heart attacks will continue claiming our loved ones long before their time.

"An aortic rupture is usually the first symptom that an aneurysm exists, even though they take years to develop. What's tragic is that detecting aortic aneurysms before they rupture is simple and costs very little."

Chapter 15

The Big Bang!

A front tire explodes and disintegrates at high speed on the highway. Blowouts can mean disaster, and they're not limited to cars and trucks. Our body has its own version, the blowout of the aorta. It's our largest artery, the mainline of life, and when it goes, it is a catastrophic event.

Stretched, weakened, thinning, and exhausted from holding back the constant pressure that drives each drop of blood around our bodies thousands of times a day for decades, it simply explodes.

The aorta itself begins at the top of the heart where it receives fast-moving, freshly-oxygenated blood ejected from the heart's left ventricle. The aorta is a tough but flexible one-inch diameter hose that extends up toward the neck. It then arches gracefully to descend through the chest into the abdomen, ultimately splitting as it continues through the pelvis and into our legs.

A rupture occurs in a weak, dilated section of the aorta called an *aneurysm*. And although the aneurysm can occur anywhere along the aorta, 95 percent of the dangerous ones occur about the level of our kidneys, above the navel but below the sternum.

Over 80 percent of its victims die quickly, many before reaching the hospital. Among those who survive to have an emergency surgical repair, nearly half die in the postoperative period. A ruptured aneurysm leaves a lot of metabolic damage in it's wake such as kidney failure, injured lungs, and brain damage. Repairing the site of the rupture isn't always enough.

An aortic rupture is usually the first symptom that an aneurysm exists, even though they take years to develop. What's tragic is that detecting aortic aneurysms before they rupture is simple and costs very little.

Unlike some other killers I'll talk about, once an aneurysm is discovered and measured, we pretty much know what to do. It is usually a matter of doing nothing or performing surgery to prevent a rupture.

This is not one of our most prolific killers, accounting for about 15,000 deaths in this country annually. But it makes the list of stupid reasons to die, because we can see it coming miles away and pick the best possible time to fix it.

A few facts: This is 85 percent a guy thing. The vast majority of ruptures are in men between sixty-five and eighty, an age range when surgical repair often makes a lot of sense. The 15 percent that attack women almost always do so *after* eighty, an age where the benefits of major surgery are not as certain.

Abdominal aortic aneurysms can be found in about 4 percent of all men over sixty-five, though most are small enough to not need treatment.

Two major causes, aside from being male, are a history of smoking *ever in their lives* and a history of high blood pressure. It also runs in families. The risk of an aortic aneurysm increases about four times for those with a close relative who had one.

A normal aorta in the abdomen is about 1.6 centimeters wide, between one-half and three-quarters of an inch. When an abnormal expansion grows beyond 3.0 cm in width, we call it an aneurysm.

The disease process is a large-scale example of hardening of the arteries, except the effects on the aorta are different. Inflammatory white blood cells still infiltrate the artery wall, weakening the structure with digesting enzymes. The aorta, however, is much too big and the blood flow too strong for a blood clot to plug its nearly one-inch diameter.

Instead, years of chronic inflammation result in loss of the tough and flexible fibers that support the aortic wall. A weak area begins to stretch under the relentless fluid pressure, and eventually a large section of the wall is pushed out of shape, much like an over-inflated balloon.

We know that smoking affects the white blood cells that are part of the atherosclerotic process, causing them to increase their production of enzymes that eat away at our artery walls, making them less elastic, thinner, more brittle. But why this process should be so susceptible to *even a tiny bit* of smoking, often in the distant past, is not known with certainty.

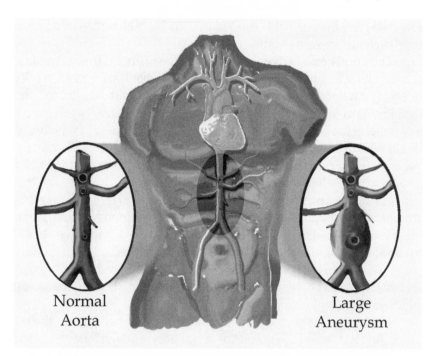

Normal Aorta   Large Aneurysm

People walk around without symptoms, completely unaware their bomb is about to detonate. They are probably also unaware we now have an incredibly simple way to find it.

On the other hand, high blood pressure's contribution to the problem is no mystery at all. The higher the pressure, the more force pushes against thin, weakened artery walls.

Once the stretching process starts, things get much worse. Basic physics states that the tension pushing outward on our ever-weakening section of aorta goes up directly with the diameter of that section. That means that when a normal 1.6 cm aorta stretches to 3.2 cm, the amount of force acting to pop that pipe has doubled. So, it's no surprise that the bigger the aneurysm, the more likely it is to burst. They usually grow beyond 5.5 cm before doing so.

Finding aortic aneurysms in the abdomen is easy. Ultrasound, the same safe and painless device that captures images of our babies in the womb, could well have been invented with aortic aneurysms in mind. It identifies fluid-fill structures such as large blood vessels with 20/20 clarity.

The test is over 96 percent sensitive and 100 percent specific, leaving virtually no doubt about who is and who is not harboring a potential time bomb. Add inexpensive, to the mix, and you've got a near-perfect screening test.

The good news is that awareness of the problem finally made it into the mainstream. Responding to evidence that screening men over age sixty-five reduces death from rupture by about 50 percent, the U.S. Preventive Services Task Force (USPSTF) recently released a recommendation for one-time screening of all men age sixty-five or higher who ever smoked. And in 2007, Medicare will actually pay for one-time screenings for both men and women who ever smoked *or* who have a relative with a history of aneurysm.

Further medical recommendations follow this one-time screening based on the clinical findings: It's recommended that small aneurysms, 3.0 cm to 3.9 cm, be ignored. Those of medium size, 4.0 cm to 5.4 cm, should be checked periodically to see how fast they grow. The big ones, 5.5 cm or wider, should be repaired right away. A fast rate of growth, more than 0.6 cm per year, should also be an indication for surgical repair.

This is a great start, because now aortic screening is on the radar of physicians and the public. But is it good enough? Is it truly the *state of the art*? I'm not convinced.

USPSTF recommendations usually result from expert, carefully weighted evaluation of all the available information regarding the screening being considered, and I think they do a good job. But their final reports address not only clinical issues but also the cost-effectiveness of screening – how much the screening will cost per life saved. And they place more importance than I do on the psychological stress that accompanies abnormal test results.

I believe the cost issue is irrelevant when dealing with informed, motivated patients, willing to pay out-of-pocket for what they decide is important. Each individual life is priceless but, as I described in Chapter 8, it's not possible or reasonable to expect government or insurance programs to pay for screening everyone for everything.

As with all screening tests, patients should be informed about the possible outcomes and what a specific result might mean before the test is given. They must be willing to accept any uncertainty in the results. In my experience, education and a strong relationship between patient and physician are excellent treatments for anxiety related to the search for potential health problems.

I have no doubt that the vast majority of ruptured aortas do indeed occur after the age of sixty-five, but my personal experience colors my view. Of the four critical aneurysms that have come my way, all but one occurred in men *under* the age of sixty.

Of the four, one died before reaching the emergency room, one survived surgical repair, (his rupture occurred only three blocks from a major hospital), and another died the day after his surgery. These three cases were before I started routine screening. The fourth patient had a 6.6-cm aneurysm found by routine ultrasound at age fifty-nine. It was successfully repaired. Since the chance of rupture of a 6.6-cm aneurysm increases by 20 percent with each passing year, he is very happy he didn't wait six years to be screened.

Widespread screening under the age of sixty-five would identify a lot of people with small aneurysms. These patients would need to be followed over time to track the growth of the aneurysms, because it is not yet known how small aneurysms are likely to behave in a younger population. But aside from this consideration and assuming an educated, willing patient, I don't see the down side of screening at a younger age.

In addition, routine abdominal ultrasound in my own practice has incidentally uncovered two early cancers of the kidney and provided a baseline "picture" for all patients which reveals individual quirks such as benign liver or kidney cysts. This baseline record can be useful for untangling any future abdominal problems. I currently recommend an ultrasound of the entire abdomen every four years for all patients forty or older.

Repairing a large or rapidly-growing aneurysm involves grafting an artificial aorta segment made of protein-lined Dacron to the inside of the weakened area. The body quickly grows a layer of beautiful endothelial cells to cover the inner surface. The blood flowing from the aorta will not know the difference.

This is a big surgery. The operation itself carries a 2 to 4 percent chance of death, so it's reserved for only big or rapidly growing aneurysms. If you need repair but don't have any symptoms such as back or groin pain, there is time to plan. Studies show that the best surgical outcomes in this case are achieved at hospitals where at least 30 such surgeries are performed every year.

There are times when major surgery can and should be performed in the comfort and support of one's hometown community hospital. This isn't one of them. You not only need a surgeon who specializes in aortic repair but a hospital that does as well. The nursing staff, the ICU team, therapists, and other specialists all need to have experience with aneurysm patients, because what happens after the surgery matters as much as a superb performance in the operating room. It's not enough to be at a top-notch surgical hospital; you specifically need one with *aortic aneurysm experience*.

Now, what if an aneurysm hasn't ruptured but the patient is experiencing pain in the back, groin, or testicles and maybe fever as well. That changes things. Time then becomes the biggest enemy, and your best chance for survival is *immediate* surgery. Any delay to transfer to a different hospital would be a foolish gamble.

Newer surgical approaches are being studied. *Endovascular repair* is a new, much less invasive procedure which places a fabric sleeve into the aorta, threading it up through the large arteries in the groin. Unlike the traditional surgery, it is not a definitive repair, but rather a means for providing *some* protective support. It acts to widen the artery *downstream* from the weakened area, thus reducing back-pressure on the aneurysm while support from the cloth sleeve itself directly relieves some of the strain on the aneurysm wall.

So far, the results are mixed. Fewer patients die from the procedure than from the major surgery, for obvious reasons, but this gain is gradually lost over time, and some of these patients eventually have a rupture. At the end of two years, the overall survival of both groups has been about the same.

At this point, I would advise a patient who is younger and not too ill for major surgery to have a complete repair with a Dacron graft at a hospital with an excellent reputation in this field.

In preparing for surgical repair of an aortic aneurysm, it's important to lower the blood pressure as much as safely possible. Doing so with the class of medications called beta blockers has been shown to drastically cut the death rate from surgical complications when taken for a week prior to surgery.

Aortic Dissection

I opened this book with an account of the tragic death of actor John Ritter, who succumbed to aortic dissection - a tear in the aorta, which is different than a full blown rupture. In dissection, the aorta is usually normal in size with no telltale bulging.

Then a plaque rupture of the inner lining allows blood to work its way between the inner and outer walls, splitting, or dissecting, the layers of the aortic wall. Unlike aortic aneurysms, aortic dissection usually occurs in the chest, not the abdomen, and can cause severe pain, sometimes mistaken for a heart attack.

Aortic dissections do not qualify as a stupid reason to die, because we don't yet have a way to predict them. But I mention them here because they are sometimes missed by physicians. Like aneurysm, they prefer to attack men, but they don't wait for us guys to get old, often striking in our forties and fifties.

Mr. Ritter's family was reported to be suing the hospital in which he died, claiming that confusion over his chest pain - they say the doctors thought he was having a heart attack - delayed the surgery he needed to save his life. I can't comment on the merits of such a case and have no idea how true these media articles are except to say that when the "chest pain hits the fan," confusion is hard to avoid.

However, recent review articles have supported the fact that once a heart attack has been "ruled out," patients with chest pain are often discharged without a close look at the aorta. After all, aortic dissection is fairly uncommon, affecting only 2 in 10,000 people while emergency rooms everywhere see a daily diet of heart attacks. And dissection can be gradual and less dramatic than an aortic rupture; the symptoms can come and go and can be quite vague.

It's an "awareness" problem - so be on your guard should you or a loved one find yourself in the emergency room experiencing chest pain with no obvious cause. It's OK to ask the physicians to evaluate for aortic disease.

What might the presence of aortic disease - aneurysm or dissection - tell us about the likelihood for other atherosclerotic problems such as heart attack? Probably a lot. Although it's possible to find a few people with aneurysm but no heart disease, and it's very common to find people with heart disease but no aneurysm, the risk factors for both overlap. Do not let the presence or absence of one form of atherosclerosis help you choose whether or not to be tested for the other! Look for both separately.

"We must consider every possible culprit, even if we already have one in custody."

Chapter 16

Not Always the Usual Suspects

Heart attacks, strokes and ruptured aneurysms all happen because of hardening of the arteries. And arteries harden for good reasons, some well-understood and others more obscure. But in most cases, we now have the ability to determine why one person's arteries develop atherosclerosis while another's do not. Even better, we can do something about it.

High cholesterol, hypertension, diabetes, smoking, and other conditions contribute to atherosclerosis. Yet, so far, I haven't been pushing the traditional practice of focusing attention on all the things that *might* cause it, practices like measuring everyone's good and bad cholesterol, blood pressure or suggesting a low-fat or low-carb or low-salt diet. These are often important things, but we must not put the cart before the horse.

First, I want to check patients for real evidence of coronary artery disease or aortic aneurysm. This is especially true in people middle-age and older, where we can expect to see a problem if it's been brewing, and where patients are old enough that the *absence* of such a problem is also meaningful.

The value of this approach is reflected in two personal cases. I personally had a stubborn cholesterol level, well over 300. My close friend, Frank, had a level of only 168. My blood pressure was also higher than his. Neither of us had diabetes or smoked.

The cards were definitely stacked in Frank's favor, while a low-fat diet and daily jogging still didn't budge my awful numbers. Then we each had a heart scan. My results scored zero. No evidence at all of coronary artery disease. Frank's score of over 3000 still holds the record in my practice for the worst coronary CT score. None of the traditional causes of heart disease could explain it.

A more extensive search, including blood tests most people never get, revealed that Frank had *several* of the more obscure risk factors. There are three very important points in these two cases.

> ▶ **People with clear risk factors, such as very high cholesterol, may not develop coronary artery disease. When treatment is based solely on risk factors, these patients live in fear of a heart attack and may take unnecessary medications.**

> ▶ **Others, like Frank, appear unlikely candidates for a heart attack based on the usual assessments, but can be headed for disaster.**

> ▶ **Most important: when trouble is suspected based on one condition, the search is *not* over. All possible causes must be evaluated.**

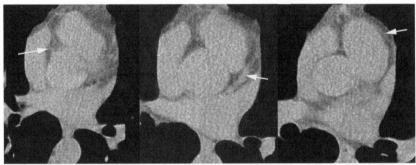

Here are samples from my EBT scan. Despite my very high cholesterol, there is no disease noted in the coronary arteries. (see arrows)

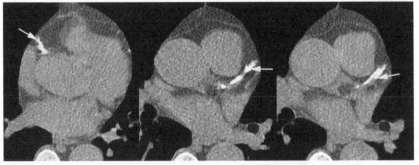

Frank's EBT scan shows extensive disease in both coronary arteries, despite normal cholesterol, blood pressure and the absence of other traditional risk factors.

If Frank's cholesterol happened to be high we might have stopped there, assuming we caught our culprit. He would have been treated only for high cholesterol. The other undiscovered problems would have continued to do damage, moving Frank closer to disaster. This happens a lot.

When we find atherosclerosis, the detective work is just beginning. We must consider every possible culprit, even if we already have one in custody. Then we need to enforce a "zero tolerance policy" by treating every condition likely to be contributing to hardening of the arteries. Aggressive treatment is the only proven way to prevent catastrophe.

So where do we start our hunt? This is where we must leave the do-it-yourself part of the prevention process behind us. The search for all likely causes of arterial disease requires a specialist in atherosclerosis management, typically a cardiologist who is using state-of-the-art methods for detecting and arresting all known risk factors.

The good news is that many cardiologists already do this for patients who survived a heart attack, artery stent placement, or coronary artery bypass surgery. These patients are at a huge risk for another "event." Their cardiologists conduct intense investigations of possible causes and provide a high level of treatment. This level of effort is known as "secondary prevention," because it's meant to prevent a second attack.

While having a very high score on an Ultra Fast heart CT isn't exactly the same as having *actually* had a heart attack, it's close enough and many cardiologists recognize this.

Of course, getting treatment to *prevent* that first heart attack is the way to go. So, no matter how much you love and trust your wonderful internist, family doctor, or nurse practitioner, if you are diagnosed with atherosclerosis, go to an expert in the disease.

Up to this point, the goal has been to get the *right* people, those whose arteries are actively hardening, under expert care. What now? It's beyond the scope of this book to present all the known causes of heart disease and the best treatments for risk. Treatment is based on the unique situation and needs of each patient. Additional information is available on my website **www.stupidreasonspeopledie.com**. But here, I can give you some important "broad strokes" of this complicated picture.

The Metabolic Syndrome

This is the biggest enemy in our war against heart disease. Metabolic Syndrome is a group of separate traits that become extra deadly when they get together. Previously known as Syndrome X and Insulin Resistance Syndrome, Metabolic Syndrome is defined by a constellation of three or more of these five conditions:

▶ **Hypertension**

▶ **High Triglycerides levels in the blood (non-cholesterol lipids)**

▶ **Low HDL cholesterol levels in the blood (HDL is known as the "good" cholesterol)**

▶ **Insulin resistance or full blown diabetes**

▶ **Truncal obesity (extra weight is carried more in the gut than on the hips)**

Each of these traits carries a statistical chance of increasing one's heart attack risk, but the combination of *any three* doubles the already substantial danger by compounding the risk of each condition. The fact is, Metabolic Syndrome is the cause of 80 percent of the heart attacks in this country. And it's very sneaky.

For example, diabetics as a group have a 25 percent shorter life span than non-diabetics. The reason is the higher rate of heart attacks and strokes in this population.

The majority of Type 2 diabetics, about 87 percent, *also* have at least two more conditions in the above list which translates into Metabolic Syndrome. It turns out that the 13 percent of diabetics *who do not have* Metabolic Syndrome are at no greater risk for heart attacks than non-diabetics! This means it isn't high blood sugar itself that causes diabetic heart disease but the Metabolic Syndrome.

Thin diabetics, without high blood pressure and with normal cholesterol and triglyceride numbers, must still control their blood sugars very carefully to avoid blindness, constant pain in their hands and feet, kidney failure, leg amputation and early death by infection. These are the ravages of high blood sugar over many years. But usually, Metabolic Syndrome gets them first, cutting short their lives even if they faithfully managed their blood sugar levels. This is all the more tragic, given that progress in preventing the other terrible complications of diabetes has exploded in recent years.

Metabolic Syndrome is on the rise. Obesity in America has grown beyond epidemic levels, more than doubling between 1990 and 2000. Only one-third of Americans *are not* overweight! One-third qualify as "obese" with a body mass index of over 30 (see Appendix 4). More than 44 percent of Americans over age fifty have Metabolic Syndrome. Think about that—nearly one-half of our population over fifty are prime candidates for an early death!

There are many different theories on why we're getting fatter and in such a deadly way. It's certainly true that we move less than we did. Heck, thanks to email and conference calling, we don't even have to walk down the hall to meet with a co-worker. What TV started in creating couch potatoes, the Internet seems to be finishing.

A diabetic expert and colleague reminded me how life has changed since the '50s. He was describing traveling in the family station wagon for summer vacation. "We'd pull into a gas station and, on rare occasion, get an amazing treat—a full 10-ounce Coke of our very own!" Today, young people often have several Big Gulps a day. In the '80s, it was the fad to run 10k's after a carbo-load the night before. Evil fat was scorned, and everyone seemed to be having no-fat frozen yogurt for lunch.

Today we still load up on carbs, but the 10k runs seem to have fallen out of style. When we don't exercise, our bodies, with million-year-old survival programming, assume we must be injured or sick. Why else would anyone lay around instead of gathering food and running away from danger?

Back in the days when our software was written, disability meant starvation and death. The body was made to react by slowing down metabolism and increasing appetite. That would allow the accumulated fat to last longer and inspire devouring food *whenever possible*, a pretty clever mechanism for surviving in the wild. We may have been cranky with hunger most of the time, but we'd survive until we were able to hunt again.

Today, the insatiable hunger from inactivity meets an *endless* food supply. The nation's weight problem is out of control and the sad thing is, once a person's weight increases, the body *does not want to let it go*. It prefers to hold onto the reserve until it's convinced you're a super athlete. Only then will it crank up its metabolism and expend a few calories.

Changes in our bodies occur when counter-regulatory systems alter the way our fat cells, muscle cells, stomach, and brain communicate with each other. They instruct the body on how to package, transport and burn sugar and fat as fuel.

This semi-permanent change is called the Metabolic Syndrome.

Forget the war on drugs and crime. The real killer is easy to find and easy to take into custody. All but one of the five conditions associated with Metabolic Syndrome can be identified with a blood test or by measuring blood pressure and tummy size. The fifth, insulin resistance, requires a glucose tolerance test with insulin levels added to the blood test.

Debate continues over the best healthcare approach to cardiovascular risks and Metabolic Syndrome in particular. Some voice concern that promoting the concept of a Metabolic Syndrome will cause physicians to focus only on its five components and ignore many other risk factors. Most experts agree insulin resistance seems to be the worst of the bunch, and that perhaps the other four risk factors are actually caused by insulin resistance.

So the name may change with time, reverting to the term *Insulin Resistance Syndrome* or changing to a brand new one like *Cardiometabolic Risk Syndrome*.

But whatever it happens to be called by the time you read this, treatment must be aggressive and, in most cases, must include weight loss. Caution: Even an effective exercise and dieting program alone is unlikely to reduce the risk. Medication will most likely be needed, especially when there is already evidence of atherosclerosis in a Metabolic Syndrome patient. Currently, the best strategy is to go after each of the known risk factors individually.

I'll share a few of my own strategies with the caveat that I am not offering you, the reader, personal advice. You are a unique individual, and I have no way to know what is in your best interests. Keep in mind as well that new information, new research, and new technology can render my current strategies obsolete at any time.

Blood Pressure

First, high blood pressure should be controlled, below the level of 130/80 and even lower if no side-effects of treatment develop. Diabetics have a powerful survival benefit just by maintaining lower blood pressure. The choice of medication matters and depends on the patient's other co-existing problems. Certain classes of drugs are well known to protect the kidneys from the ravages of diabetes and hypertension while others help a damaged heart survive.

It's a complex decision process, often involving strategic combinations, but a specialist should have no trouble explaining his or her recommendations. After several years of successful blood pressure control, along with an established program of weight loss and exercise, it may be possible to reduce or even discontinue blood pressure medications.

When the disease processes that cause Metabolic Syndrome are under control, the arteries can actually heal and return to normal functioning, bringing self regulation of blood pressure back down to a lower level.

Cholesterol Management

Cholesterol management is a huge subject. It must be specifically tailored according to each patient's profile.

First, a little background. Cholesterol and other lipids do not travel freely in the bloodstream. Water and oil do not mix. Our cholesterol is packaged into water-soluble particles called Lipoprotein Complexes. These particles also contain special enzymes and structures that help cells recognize and exchange lipids with them.

The particles that deliver lipids to our tissues happen to be of low density and so are termed Low-Density Lipoprotein Cholesterol, or LDL Cholesterol. You may have also heard LDL described as the "bad cholesterol," because high blood levels of LDL seem to be correlated with more heart risk. I'd describe them as a leaky dump truck, getting the job done but making a mess along the way.

Higher density particles, termed High Density Lipoprotein Cholesterol, or HDL, also carry lipids but have a different set of proteins. They bring cholesterol and other lipids from the body tissues *back* to the liver for recycling. They are the efficient street sweepers, collecting lipids and leaving the route cleaner. That's why HDL is considered the "good cholesterol."

Many people know about the dangers of bad cholesterol and benefits of good cholesterol. Remember, a low level of the good cholesterol is one of the elements in Metabolic Syndrome.

When atherosclerosis is clearly present, a *statin* medication is used to lower LDL cholesterol, but it will also help decrease inflammation in the arterial plaques, offering a two-for-one benefit. For this reason, statins form the foundation of current cholesterol treatment. But this is only the first layer of treatment that many patients need, because good and bad cholesterol aren't the only problem.

Nature has a few wily tricks up her sleeve that fool us if we rely only on a basic lipid analysis. The lipids have a greater story to tell. A patient can have a high level of the "good" cholesterol only to find out, after the heart attack, that they weren't all that great. Certain genetic traits can leave the cholesterol "street sweepers" defective. The body senses cholesterol isn't returning to the liver as it should and responds by producing *more* defective HDL. The HDL level is high, but it is doing a lousy job.

A similar event happened to Frank, my same friend who holds the dubious "World's Worst Heart Scan" trophy. He had a perfectly normal total cholesterol (168) and a nice low LDL subset (98). But not all LDL particles are alike. Some are big, some small. Some are "oxidized," some are not.

When people walk around with most of their LDL particles of the small and oxidized variety, macrophage cells patrolling our coronary arteries say "yum!" and gorge on this molecular fast food, getting fat and stuck, creating new plaque. And, unlike many well-controlled systems in our bodies that know when they've had enough, the macrophages never get full, devouring every oxidized LDL snack that comes their way.

Frank's other problem was a genetic one. His LDL particles had a protein attachment, called a kringle, that made his LDL look and perhaps behave like one of the proteins that help our blood clot. This is called Lipoprotein [a], pronounced "LP little a" (See Appendix 5).

Special labs, like the Berkeley Heart Lab in California, are able to measure properties such as the size and oxidation state of cholesterol particles. Genetic studies help profile some of the proteins, such as apoprotein E (apoE), that travel with our cholesterol particles and, if mutated, might cause them to be defective, unable to perform their functions efficiently.

Armed with this more complete information, a specialist can recommend treatments targeted at these specific problems. They may use medications known as "fibrates" and possibly high doses of the vitamin B3, Niacin.

One brief aside: Although you can buy Niacin over the counter, PLEASE do not take this drug or give it to anyone else without the recommendation of a physician. At the doses needed to be helpful, it has more side-effects than almost any other medication I prescribe. Just because it's a vitamin doesn't mean it's harmless. For certain patients it is a life saver, but it's not pleasant to take and requires close monitoring by a physician.

Exciting new medications are in the development pipeline that address these special problems and are eagerly anticipated in the medical community. Our hope is they will enhance already-effective treatments for preventing heart attacks and strokes while being kinder and gentler than drugs like Niacin.

Insulin Resistance And Diabetes

When I started medical practice, I hated dealing with two seemingly hopeless conditions: diabetes and back pain. I often still dread the challenge of treating a bad back, but time has kindly advanced the management of diabetes. Unsung heroes, brilliant scientists behind the medical scene, have advanced our knowledge about the disease and spurred development of tremendous new technology for its treatment.

As a result of their tools, I consider myself top notch in the treatment of Diabetes and Insulin Resistance, now my favorite area of patient care. The progress in this field reminds me of the revolutions in the computer industry; it seems exponential. In this case, the revolution in diabetic management was created by the pharmaceutical industry.

As I mentioned before, Metabolic Syndrome afflicts most type 2 diabetics, causes semi-permanent changes in the set point for the body's weight, appetite, and in the utilization of fat and glucose for fuel, all leading to a beer gut, chronic hunger, widespread inflammation in the body, and, too often, early death.

Treatment for diabetes began with animal insulin shots, then moved to medications that flogged the already exhausted insulin-secreting cells to secrete even more. But unlike type 1 diabetes, which usually strikes children by suddenly wiping out these cells, type 2 diabetes is not about insulin, at least not for the first ten or twenty years. It's about the tissues, liver, muscle, and adipose, that are *supposed* to sense and respond to the body's insulin by taking in and storing glucose from the bloodstream. Eventually, these tissues grow insensitive to the insulin signal. The body responds by "shouting" at them with higher and higher levels of insulin.

Years before blood sugar rises, the body's insulin system kicks into overdrive, trying to keep glucose levels normal but bathing our insides with high insulin concentrations. High levels of insulin are bad. They cause atherosclerosis and probably represent a major contribution to the death rate from Metabolic Syndrome.

New drugs, known as insulin sensitizers, are now available to address insulin resistance directly. Glucophage, Actos, and Avandia have all been shown to delay the onset of diabetes and decrease the rate of early death. I use them a lot. Still, until 2005, there was nothing that could reverse the deadly changes that kept Metabolic Syndrome patients fat and hungry. That's changing.

Brand new treatment approaches, at the time of this writing, are targeting the neuroendocrine changes of Metabolic Syndrome. One drug, exenatide (Byetta), mimics a naturally-occurring hormone in the body, GLP-1, which not only controls blood sugar more effectively but also contributes to significant weight loss in overweight diabetics. Many of these patients lose 60 pounds or more in under a year without hunger pains. They often feel more energized and happier, not just because of the weight loss but as a direct result of a medication that restores healthier metabolic functioning.

There is preliminary evidence that it may also slow down the inevitable burnout of the beta cells that makes even type 2 diabetics eventually require insulin. It doesn't work perfectly for everyone, but it helps most of my patients who've tried it.

Another drug from the same class, pramlintide (Symlin), is for diabetics who already require insulin shots. It also mimics a natural hormone, amylin, that helps "tell" patients they are full. Natural amylin is meant to be released along with insulin after a meal. But in insulin-dependent diabetics, amylin, like insulin, is no longer released from the beta cells.

Many more medications of this class of drugs, known as the incretins, will no doubt join our toolbox in the next few years, targeting the disease process of Metabolic Syndrome right at its core.

Not yet on the market in this country, is the first of another new class of medicines that target the endocannabinoid system. This newly explored system plays a huge role in hunger and in the unhealthy use of body fuels that define the Metabolic Syndrome.

The name is no coincidence. This is the system that is triggered by marijuana to cause the munchies. A new drug, rimonabant (Acomplia), hits the same receptors, the CB1 receptors, but has the opposite effect. Already released in France, the preliminary results show that not only does the patient experience less craving for food, but also for cigarettes and alcohol. It turns out that CB1 receptors exist not only in our brains but in our fat tissue as well. The abnormal use of our body's fuel, the high triglycerides, the low HDLs, and the chronically-high levels of inflammation, all typical of the Metabolic Syndrome, are directly reversed by this medication.

The hope is we will reverse the spiral of weight gain, hunger, and more weight gain, which fuels the Metabolic Syndrome, and eventually restore a more normal metabolic system, reducing the need for so many medications.

It isn't a matter of simple willpower when the body's chemistry is in control of weight gain. When the body says you must be a certain weight, *that* is where your weight will go. Medications that provide a normal sense of satiety and well-being inspire better eating habits and a more active lifestyle. We will watch for side-effects of this new class of medicine, which appears to affect mood or pleasure centers as well as metabolism. But for smokers, alcoholics or the obese, the greatest threat is the drug they are addicted to: tobacco, alcohol, or food. And for the diabetic, the greatest threat is Metabolic Syndrome.

One last point about weight loss in Metabolic Syndrome: it is not necessary to lose *all* the excess weight to see improvement in the syndrome. Turning the direction around from gaining to losing is what counts. Eight pounds off a 200-pound person makes a big difference in the severity of the damage done. It's also common for a patient starting an exercise program or medication to see a decrease in inches around their waist before there's a drop on the scale, and this shift is a very good sign.

We've talked about a few of the culprits that are associated with atherosclerosis. The current list includes the following conditions— some obviously guilty, some still under suspicion:

- ▶ **hypertension**
- ▶ **high LDL cholesterol**
- ▶ **low HDL cholesterol**
- ▶ **diabetes**
- ▶ **insulin resistance**
- ▶ **small, dense highly oxidized LDL**
- ▶ **high VLDL with high triglycerides**
- ▶ **apoprotein E mutation**
- ▶ **elevated C-Reactive Protein (hs-CRP)**
- ▶ **elevated homocysteine**
- ▶ **elevated LP[a]**
- ▶ **elevated interleukin 6**
- ▶ **elevated fibrinogen**
- ▶ **elevated plasminogen activator inhibitor-1 (PAI-1)**
- ▶ **dysfunctional HDL (low HDL 2b subset)**

. . . and more to come as new information emerges.

This is why it makes sense to do the most extensive searches *after* finding an atherosclerosis problem. That's not to say people shouldn't be checked for risk factors before middle age.

Obesity and it's frequent companion, type 2 diabetes, is occurring in younger and younger people every year. The term "adult-onset diabetes" was abandoned when type 2 diabetes began appearing in obese children as young as six. Although alarming new studies have sometimes found significant amounts of coronary plaque in obese *adolescent children*, it usually takes years before a young person develops enough atherosclerosis to be seen with a scan. So physicians should keep watch for the obviously guilty risk factors in overweight kids, especially those contributing to Metabolic Syndrome. In fact, state-of-the-art care is now based on early intervention in children to *head off* full blown Metabolic Syndrome. Once again, it may be decades before the standard of care catches up.

Diet, exercise, adequate rest, balance in our work and family lives, all matter a great deal, and you'll find thousands of books dedicated to healthier lifestyles. But right now, this minute, more than one hundred million Americans have heart disease, cerebrovascular disease, or an aortic aneurysm preparing to rupture.

Our most immediate concern must be to control the runaway perpetrator—atherosclerosis.

Next up, the big 'C.'

~~~

Killing Cancer

There is something enormously satisfying when a relentless killer becomes a hunted fugitive. I relish that satisfaction every time we capture another cancer.

I imagine the sneaky invader hiding silently, determined not to be discovered until it is big enough to overpower its victim, only to have its quiet, malignant existence exploded as we rip it out of its comfortable lair and plunge it into a smelly jar of formaldehyde.

Some cancers are easy to find, some are not. Some can be cured if found early, some can't. Some we know how to prevent, most we do not. But there is a small gang responsible for the majority of cancer deaths, and we can do a lot to stop them.

We're going to talk about the most prolific cancer killers, each of which must be found early, before it takes over. Today, using the state-of-the-art in early detection will be our most important weapon.

I'll start with the cancer that, as far back as I can remember, holds the title of *Cancer Public Enemy Number One*.

~~~

"Feeling whole again is just one cigarette away. So is returning to a pack-a-day habit."

Chapter 17

Smoking Out the King

Hail the King. You've got to hand it to a cancer that kills more people than all the others combined. The lung cancer death toll keeps going up, about 164,000 U.S. deaths per year as I write this.

Smoking accounts for 90 percent of them. The other 10 percent occurring in non-smokers reminds us that lung cancer was here long before cigarettes. However, we humans, with a lot of help from tobacco, get the credit for making it the undisputed King.

And that's a shame. Because smoking is great. It takes some getting used to, but once you get past the burnt ash taste and let the combination of nicotine and Zen-breathing kick in, it's a wonderful way to spend ten minutes.

I have never seen a driver with road-rage gun his engine, then flip off and cut in on another driver while inhaling tobacco. The worst I've witnessed is a guy *too* relaxed, dawdling in front of me at half the speed limit. This can put me in an angry snit, provoking me to gun my engine, flip him off and zip in front of him.

Cigarettes may prevent nasty blowups, angry outbursts, car crashes, maybe even manslaughter. They can enhance the aftermath of romance, promote quiet introspection or provide much-needed escape from pressure or boredom. They sooth the contemporary savage beast in many ways.

Then, of course, there's the down side:

If you smoke, you will most likely die much younger than you would otherwise. The habit turns ugly in the form of heart attack, stroke, suffocation from emphysema, or lung cancer that spreads throughout your body. Before then, you may need to have your

gangrenous feet cut off when blood flow no longer reaches your
lower limbs.

One or two cigarettes a day are all it takes to triple your
long-term risk for stroke or heart attack. Just one single puff
can actually set off either event. Plus, society will now treat you
like a child murderer.

The End.

I don't actually think of smoking as a stupid reason people die. A
stupid reason for dying, in my mind, is one that is easily avoided or
which results from missing an easy opportunity to identify a problem
early and treat it effectively.

There is nothing easy about giving up a smoking habit. Every
smoker in civilized society knows how dangerous it is, knows they are
playing with fire. They are not ignorant or defiant or actively trying to
die a horrible death. They pay their money, take their chances, and
light up for a reason.

Who would choose to rot their lungs and arteries, to be treated as
second-class citizens, to smell like an ashtray, and put out nearly five
bucks a pack if there wasn't a huge psychological benefit from smoking?

Many believe that nicotine addiction is the reason people don't
quit. It's not. It's a rare smoker who can't get past the physical
dependency on nicotine. It only lasts a few days and, for most smokers, the physical addiction isn't that powerful. A minority of smokers
is truly addicted physically—the ones who light their first cigarette of
the day *before* setting foot out of bed. For them, being deprived of
nicotine throughout the night is almost too much too bear. For these
folks, the first day of giving up smoking is a shock to their system.

But most people who try to quit pull it off for at least a few days,
often for two or three weeks, sometimes for months, before going
back to smoking. After the first week, the nicotine withdrawal, and,
therefore, the physical dependency, is completely over.

So, if the physical addiction itself is not the culprit, why do they
start again? For the same reason an alcoholic falls off the wagon or a
heroin addict goes through the hell of withdrawal, only to get hooked
again: *because it fills a genuine need.*

Nonsmokers may not understand or appreciate what those needs
are, but we don't have to. Instead, we need to support every new
approach and each and every effort a smoker makes to stop.

The average successful former smoker got there only after trying to quit, and failing, at least six times. That's six *real* times, quitting for months, until they have "just one" cigarette at a party.

Failed attempts to quit should be applauded because the *attempt* is essential to their eventual success. Focusing on the failure only delays the next important attempt.

I've heard quitting described by dozens of patients as losing a piece of themselves, like an arm, a leg, or a loved one. Anthony put it this way, "Imagine you lost your wife (he had), and the emptiness doesn't let up. But in *this* case, at the back of your mind you always know that by giving in and doing something you shouldn't, you could feel whole again just one more time. Of course it's not as bad as losing *her*, doc, but it's the same kind of feeling."

Feeling whole again is just one cigarette away. So is returning to a pack-a-day habit. Is there anything else that can fill that void?

Nicotine replacement in gum, patches, or inhalers can help break the quitting process down into more manageable steps. The drug bupropion, known as Wellbutrin or Zyban, can decrease the urge in some people, about twenty percent of those who try it. As I write this, new medications are being developed that directly block receptors in the brain which promote smoking, alcoholism *and* overeating. And a new medication, varenicline, (Chantix) has just been released to block nicotine receptors, taking the joy out of smoking.

The previously mentioned drug, rimonabant, (Accomplia) not yet available in the U.S., helps treat obesity and Metabolic Syndrome and also curbs tobacco cravings. At this moment, a new vaccine, in clinical trials, is being used to stimulate the production of antibodies against nicotine. It turns out that sticking an antibody onto a nicotine molecule prevents it from reaching the brain and exerting its addictive effect.

In my practice, I have been known to go out on a limb for some highly motivated folks, providing short-term prescriptions for *other* habit-forming drugs, like tranquilizers, to decrease the emotional anguish they feel when they first quit. My logic goes like this: There is almost nothing I could prescribe to any smoker that would come close to the toxicity or addictive risk of a cigarette. If it gets them off tobacco, it's worth it. Obviously, I monitor these patients very closely.

What, short of a deadly illness, can help motivate a smoker to quit? We have seen how the heart scan reveals hardening of the arteries. The same type of scan can also expose emphysema of the lungs, long before the smoker truly feels its effects. Abnormal scans can be big motivators for quitting. It is one thing to accept the abstract possibility of death by smoking; it's something altogether different to actually *see* the reality of tobacco's effects. Once revealed as a concrete threat, people are more motivated to take action.

If you don't smoke, don't start.

If you do, quitting is worth the effort. Getting the necessary help to quit should be the number one to-do on your healthcare agenda. Really. Number one.

All other health screenings, state-of-the-art therapies, meditation, exercise, macrobiotic diets, and good clean living cannot begin to offset the danger from smoking. Giving them priority over quitting is like worrying about your car's tire pressure, grade of oil, or air freshener while you're stalled on a railroad track hearing a whistle in the distance.

It's the big-ticket killers that matter, and smoking is the biggest ticket of all. It increases the already-high risk for heart attack and stroke by three times and the risk of lung cancer by ten. It suffocates with emphysema, sends blood clots to the lungs, and increases the odds of breast, bladder, esophageal, and other cancers.

If you've failed before, try again. Quitting *is* possible. Not easy, but *possible*. Don't hesitate to demand help from friends, co-workers, and loved ones. If your spouse smokes, the least they can do is smoke *away* from you, and it's so much better if you quit together.

A real friend will support your efforts, not sabotage you with kindness. "Oh, you can have just one with me; you've earned it," or with guilt, "You're no fun now." Non-supportive friends may mean it's time to look for new ones. That's often what it takes.

Don't be too proud to use medication if your physician recommends it. For many highly motivated people, it's not just about willpower. Besides, it's not like you're drug free. Modern pharmacology would be hard pressed to come up with a more toxic drug than just one more cigarette per day. Remember, the risk of *not* taking needed medications is often hundreds of times higher than of taking them. This is a no-brainer when it comes to quitting tobacco.

Some believe that once they've smoked for a long while, it does little good to quit. Not true. Smokers who quit for more than 15 years have an 80 to 90 percent reduction in risk of lung cancer compared to people who continue to smoke.

On the other hand, the person who develops a fatal lung cancer often does quit after the terrifying discovery. One might ask, "Why bother?" but quit they do. The tragedy is that they discover the ability to quit was there all along; they just didn't have the motivation, faith, or the support they needed for success.

Screening for Lung Cancer

Is it possible to find lung cancer early and often enough to make a dent in the death rate? We don't know yet, but we will soon.

At present, the only thing ever proven to lower the death rate from lung cancer, beyond the rare surgical cure, is to not smoke in the first place. Studies looking at how an annual chest x-ray affects the survival from lung cancer show that the eventual death rate is the same. It appeared that lung cancer patients who received screening x-rays lived a year longer, on average, than those who didn't. But that's just because the discovery of their tumor occurred about a year earlier with the x-ray picture. The actual outcomes were the same for both groups.

In such a situation, I might prefer not to get the chest x-ray. I'd die on the same day but would know death was coming for an extra year. If there's no hope, give me ignorance for as long as possible.

Newer screening, however, holds the promise of a truly longer life for some lung cancer victims. The same high-speed CT scan machines that show us diseased coronary arteries can find lung tumors at sizes smaller than ever before. Follow-up tests, such as a positron emission tomography scan or PET Scan, can show whether a suspicious lung nodule is using glucose at a higher rate than normal, so an informed decision can be made about if and when to operate to remove suspicious growths.

Time will tell if we can significantly lower the death rate of lung cancer through widespread screening, detecting the tumor early enough to stop its metastatic spread. But just at the time of this writing, the International Early Lung Cancer Action Program, I-ELCAP, has published the results of a twelve-year, 31,000-patient study that demonstrated a ten-year survival rate of over 80 percent in lung cancer patients who underwent CT screening. The ten-year survival rate without screening is a miserable 5 percent! Visit **www.ielcap.org** for details.

Of some concern is the possibility that many smokers, reflecting human behavior, will interpret a normal scan of their lungs as an all-clear invitation to keep smoking. It wouldn't take a big percentage of screened patients who continued smoking from an irrational and very false sense of security, to negate any progress in survival from early detection. On the other hand, one small study suggests that screening actually leads to a higher quit rate in smokers, regardless of the test findings. As always, any meaningful screening should be accompanied by personalized and complete patient education before testing is performed.

Again, if you smoke, stop. That might be a full-time job for a while so treat it like one. Look into every known source of success you can find. Try them all, several times if necessary. They say "what you focus on expands," and in this case it is certainly true. The more you focus on quitting, the more often you attempt it, with new resolve, medications, nicotine gum, acupuncture, herbs, new friends, or moving to Tibet, the more likely you are to succeed.

If you love a smoker, share this information with them and support them if they choose to quit, even if they fail again and again.

If you currently smoke or have been a past smoker of ten or more pack-years *(pack-years is the number of years one smokes multiplied by the average number of packs smoked each day-two packs a day for ten years is twenty pack-years, as is one pack a day for twenty years)* you may wish to consider a high-resolution CT scan of your lungs. I've had several friends and patients discover very early lung tumors, but only time will tell if they will survive to beat lung cancer in the end. Screening looks very promising, but for now, lung cancer is still the King.

"Among all the deadly cancers, it is the slowest and laziest. It should have no chance of killing a single person in a country as fortunate as ours."

Chapter 18

The *Real* Story of the Tortoise and the Hare

The tortoise in the original story is an inspirational character, plodding along at a steady pace to win the race. The cancer that invades the colon also plods along, patiently focused on its objective.

I'll give away the ending. He's a tortoise gone bad, his inspiration is death. And many of us rabbits, who could easily take him, let him get to the finish line way ahead of us.

Here's the thing: colon cancer is a *moron*. Among all the deadly cancers, it is the slowest and laziest. It should have *no* chance of killing a single person in a country as fortunate as ours. But it does. While our healthcare system debates what to pay for, and patients delay screening because of the cost or the indelicate nature of the procedure, the tortoise lumbers along unnoticed.

It starts as a slow-growing, low-grade but obvious tumor, a pre-cancerous polyp. It takes years to grow into an aggressive, high-grade killer, so it's easy to underestimate, even disregard. It gets a significant head start, and by the time we notice, the outcome is a given. Race over. Tortoise one, patient zero.

One trick of the tortoise is to pick a path we don't like to have examined. Its other trick is to keep a low profile, providing no sign or symptom until we're in deep trouble.

We have many years during which we can find and cure this deadly cancer *during* the screening procedure, without so much as a pin prick to our skin, never mind major surgery, radiation, or chemotherapy. Failing that, there's a window of time when it can be cured with an operation alone. But if no one is looking for it, the disease process gets too far ahead to be overtaken. By the time it shows its true colors, there's nothing we can do.

This is not a "man's disease" as many seem to believe. Women, who also must deal with risk from breast and cervical cancer, don't get a break from colon cancer. It's a 50-50 split between guys and gals. About 1 percent to 2 percent of adults get colon cancer, and about half of them will die from it. Recent statistics report about 120,000 new cases per year, about 60,000 deaths in the U.S. And most of these deaths are completely unnecessary.

Nobody, myself included, likes to look for a problem that requires entrance through the rear end or the process of getting rid of any and all poop in your intestines. But like poop, colon cancer happens. Most of us know someone who has it or who died from it.

Unlike other types of screening that require little more than a blood or urine sample, or reclining on a table for a five-minute scan, this one requires a bit of time, effort, nerve, and perhaps some hard cash. So, convincing patients to have a colonoscopy is often a hard sell. The fact is, the procedure is virtually painless, as is the preparation and aftermath.

Colon cancer typically starts as a polyp, a punching bag-shaped growth coming off the inner wall of the large intestine. Part of the polyp, the center of the bag, gradually degenerates into abnormal, *somewhat* malignant cells, and over time these cells multiply into more and more *aggressive,* malignant cells.

At some point, many of these cancers begin to leak a little blood. I don't mean the bright red blood occasionally on the tissue after a bowel movement. That usually comes from internal hemorrhoids, and although it shouldn't be ignored, it seldom comes from cancer. The blood from colon cancer isn't usually noticeable. It is picked up by chemically testing a stool sample.

Meanwhile, our determined little tumor grows down the polyp stalk and around the circumference of the inner wall of the colon, and eventually begins to obstruct passage through it.

At this point there are finally symptoms, years after the damn thing could have been discovered and easily eliminated from the race. Now, the patient is faced with the possibility the cancer has spread.

This scenario happens so often. The vast majority of people do not get screened for this cancer at all, and those who do may not get *state-of-the-art* technology.

The standard of care has long been inadequate in colon cancer screening. For decades we've been pussy-footing around with the "cost-effective" techniques of sampling stool multiple times and chemically testing it for blood, hoping that if the patient has a cancer brewing we'll get lucky and catch a bit of blood mixed with the stool. Too indirect, too often done incorrectly, and usually detecting blood from hemorrhoids, not from cancer. In my opinion, a waste of time.

An inexpensive exam, the flexible sigmoidoscopy, is a short, more primitive version of colonoscopy that was often "allowed" by insurance companies since no anesthesia is needed and, instead of a specialist, the primary care physician can usually be trained to perform the test. Just a couple of problems. Flex Sig, as it's nicknamed, only looks at one-third of the colon. And it *hurts*. I had one and *only* one.

Colonoscopy, on the other hand is the gold standard of colon cancer screening. It's a six-foot long hose with a video camera on the business end as well as a light source, ports through which to pass surgical instruments and water for rinsing the lens, and complex controls to bend and guide it. It is used to view every square inch of the colon.

And that colon must be clean. The preparation is a very thorough, osmotic laxative that will keep you close to home the day or night before your test. It isn't painful; you'll just want to be close to your bathroom. You will also have to give up eating anything other than juice, Jell-O and broth.

The patient undergoing colonoscopy is sedated, because there's no need to feel the scope as it travels through your intestine. You won't be under deep anesthesia, just in a "twilight sleep" with an intravenous narcotic and sedative. Sometimes you can watch the video screen during the procedure, but you probably won't remember it.

The colonoscopy gives a direct look at the entire colon and allows the doctor to take painless biopsy samples of any suspicious areas. Even better, if the doctor finds any polyps, he or she can usually remove them right then and there.

Because anesthesia is used, and high-tech equipment and special training are required, the procedure is only performed in hospitals or specially-equipped procedure centers. Possible danger from the procedure includes bleeding and a minute, but serious risk of perforating the colon itself. That would make a surgical repair necessary. It's important to choose highly experienced physicians to perform your test. Colonoscopy also costs more than having a mole removed in the doctor's office, between one and two thousand dollars.

Historically, insurance companies and Medicare would only pay for it if patients had symptoms, usually too late in the game, or if there was a strong family history of colon cancer.

Newer imaging technology, similar to ultra-fast CT scanning used for screening of heart disease, may soon offer an optional and less-invasive method of screening at an earlier age.

I don't support the use of this yet, because any suspicious finding means that a colonoscopy must be performed anyway. That means another procedure, another bowel prep. CT and MRI imaging technology have a way to go before they can safely replace colonoscopy, but I've learned not to underestimate the bright men and women who make such things possible.

Screening colonoscopy is gradually becoming more and more accepted by insurance plans. That's nice, I guess, but insurance or not, every man and woman needs a colonoscopy when they turn 50. Many people need them earlier. Recommendations vary, depending on which of the following groups you find yourself in:

Group 1: A person with no family history of colon cancer and a person who also has no history of colon polyps or cancer. This applies only to people with reasonably complete knowledge about their biological family and whose family members have lived reasonably long lives. This group needs their first colonoscopy no later than at age 50. If all is normal, it's probably safe to go 6 to 10 years before retesting. Remember, this cancer is slow to grow. If a polyp is found, it's usually removed at the time of the test and sent to the pathologist. Some are harmless, hyperplastic polyps, but others, adenomatous polyps and a few other types, mean your colon is trying hard to misbehave and needs close attention in the future.

Group 2: A person who has had a close relative, brother, sister, parent or grandparent, with colon cancer or polyps. Or a person who doesn't know much about their biological family, or who lost their close relatives at young ages due to accidents or other illness. Remember, having *no* family history of a disease because close family members are unknown, as in adoption, or they didn't live long enough to risk getting the disease is not the same as having a *negative* family history of the disease. People in Group 2 should have a colonoscopy at age 40.

Group 3: A person who has unexplained symptoms, such as anemia suggestive of blood loss, or other symptoms related to their intestines, such as pain, new constipation, or diarrhea, or persistent narrow caliber of stool should get the test immediately. Although the problem is likely something other than cancer, time matters a lot if cancer is present.

Group 4: A person who has been through the test before and was found to have polyps needs to be followed up regularly, every two or three years, as recommended by their physician. People who grow polyps *grow more polyps* and, if ignored, these will turn into cancer eventually. They are easily removed during colonoscopy, and regular scoping will remove these very high-risk patients from colon cancer's hit list.

Group 5: A person who has already had colon cancer needs to remain "in the system." You know who you are. You may be terrified to go back and let them look again after undergoing surgery and perhaps other wretched treatments. But screening is needed to find any *brand new polyps,* which will be a lot easier to remove than the cancer already treated. Having had cancerous polyps, you're at higher risk to have it again.

Loving Your Gut

It *might* be possible to lower your risk of colon cancer. But please don't think for one second that acting in a preventive manner gets you or your loved ones off the hook for screening. Get screened on time, because we know of nothing else that lowers your risk very much.

Conventional wisdom has long claimed that a low-fat, high-fiber diet will lower your risk of colon cancer. However, as I write this, the all-important *prospective studies* designed to look at this claim are not showing any effect of dietary fat on colon cancer risk, and the jury is still out on the cancer-reducing effects of fiber.

The fountain-of-youth claims for overpriced antioxidant supplements are nonsense. They have never been shown to have any effect at all. I'm not saying that nothing in our diet can lower the risk of colon cancer. I am saying that nothing has yet been proven to do so. It may turn out that genetics are vastly more important than diet in causing colon cancer, and I have no idea how to change what is passed on to us from our families.

Having said that, there is a lot more to the health of the colon than preventing cancer.

Our epidemic low-fiber diets are almost certain to contribute to two other colon problems: hemorrhoid vein inflammation and diverticulitis. Fiber therapy clearly helps to treat these problems in many people. When I say fiber in this context, I generally mean the part of a plant that cannot be absorbed through our digestive tract. It's typically made out of carbohydrate molecules joined together in such a way that we just can't break them apart (cellulose), and they remain far too large to pass through the intestinal wall and into our bodies. Because they are carbohydrates, they hold water like a sponge (picture gelatin that cannot be digested), and this is important for the health of our colon.

Over the last 10,000 years or so, man has evolved food preparation into a high art form. Thank you ancestors! The only catch is that in the process we have seriously altered our natural diet. After all, there is nothing actually natural about bread or cheese, or cooking for that matter. We've been "processing" our food for millennia, refining and improving flavors and textures. I'm thrilled about it, but the superb quality of our meals comes at the expense of removing most of that indigestible fiber from our diet.

Our native diet was probably closer to that of a bushman: fruit, nuts, roots, vegetables, bugs, and the occasional animal. Our bodies were designed around predominantly raw plants, so our colon expects a certain amount of indigestible fiber. It relies upon it to function efficiently. Today, we extract and concentrate the nutritional parts of food, the starch, sugars, fats, proteins, and use them alone. Early man didn't use vegetable oil, white flour, granulated sugar, cheese, or sweet creamery butter. These products represent a lot of fiber-less nutrition, so a modern diet means a dramatic drop in the average amount of fiber per calorie.

Bread might be the best thing to happen to our palate, but it's a disaster to our large intestines. Tortillas, French bread, Pita bread, Nan bread, Sponge bread, Bagels, Pasta, Noodles, white rice, you name it, a version of concentrated starch for every culture. Humans relish it. Fat, too, is used in every form possible from olive oil to ice cream. Even salads are smothered in dressings that contain most of the calories on the plate.

The result of eating these foods means we get very little fiber, and the colon winds up with stool that is more concentrated than it was meant to handle. Aside from the obvious, there are some nasty things in the stool. One is a molecule called superoxide. This byproduct of colon chemistry has a nasty habit of destroying other molecules through oxidation—the act of stealing electrons from other "victim" molecules. Such compounds, in high concentrations, wear out the lining of the colon faster than necessary. They require a higher rate of cell division to supply young replacements for damaged cells. However, we only get a finite number of cell divisions before the copies accrue too many mistakes to work properly. In other words, a concentrated stool ages our colon prematurely.

Fiber bulks up the size of the stool with "solid water," allowing noxious molecules to spread into a larger volume, thereby becoming more diluted. When it comes to poop, dilution is a good thing. Think of accidentally splashing concentrated bleach on your clothes. First you get a white spot and, after a washing or two, you are left with a hole through the fabric. Yet, when you dilute bleach with enough water, it's safe to wash your clothes in it. Dilution slows chemical reactions.

Another property of fiber is that it makes things move through your system faster. This cuts down the time that your colon is exposed to irritants. One main function of the colon is to reabsorb most of the water that is pumped into your digestive tract. For that reason, the stool is most solid near the "end of the line," in the sigmoid and rectum where it sits and waits to evacuate. This is thought to be one of the reasons that more colon cancers occur in this area.

I have no intention of cutting down on Mexican food, and I'm not one bit tempted to dine on steamed bugs. On the other hand, a bran muffin and daily salad are a good start, but they aren't enough. The simplest way I know to fix the problem is to take a daily supplement of pure fiber. Added to your regular diet, it helps even the score in the calorie/fiber ratio. One of the most widely studied supplements is psyllium husk (one brand name for this is Metamucil). Mixed with a glass of water and chugged down once or twice daily, it does a lot to restore balance to your system. There are other types of fiber supplements available, some that provide a variety of fiber types. Time will tell which is the best choice. For now, I suggest that my patients take the one they find most agreeable.

It's not surprising that fiber is the treatment of choice for several diseases of the colon. Just as too much sun causes skin cancer, it also causes wrinkles, freckles, and many other skin abnormalities. The same applies to low-fiber diets. The risk for cancer *might* be greater, but the risk for hemorrhoid disease and diverticulitis most certainly are. Diverticula are little pockets, like caves, that form in the inner lining of the colon throughout our lives. They tend to be a trap for things like seeds, nuts and corn kernel husks, causing painful infection and even deadly perforations of the intestine that can spill infected stool into our bellies.

It has been convincingly demonstrated that fiber prevents the growth of new diverticula and helps clean out existing ones. It also helps prevent thrombosis, blood clots, within the specialized veins in the rectum called hemorrhoids.

Finally, as of this writing, there is strong evidence that a whole aspirin, 325 mg, every day might be associated with lowered colon cancer risk. I recommend daily aspirin for many patients, but the evidence of cancer prevention is not yet definitive. Taking aspirin every day is not without potential for harm, so it should be part of a deliberate health strategy developed with your doctor.

There you have it. Thwarting colon cancer is almost effortless. Show up for a colonoscopy every decade or so. Maybe add fiber to your glass of water every day to prevent other problems. If you do these two things, your odds of staying ahead of the tortoise are excellent.

Colon cancer is the second most common cancer killer in both men and women. If the obstacles you have to getting scoped are your butt, your pride, or your wallet, get over them. This is such a common disease, yet so easy to cure, which means for most people colon cancer qualifies as a really stupid reason for dying.

"This cancer doesn't play by the usual rules.
Find it early, destroy it, save a life.
That's how it's supposed to work, right?"

Chapter 19

This One Doesn't Play Fair

The #3 cancer killer of men, prostate cancer, seems to be everywhere. One in five U.S. guys develops it during their lifetime, flooding the medical system with over 230,000 new cases every year. However, only 30,000 of these men will actually die from it. Does that mean modern medicine can claim credit for curing the other 200,000 victims each year? Not really.

This cancer has been a tough one to figure out. The fact is, we've become *very good* at finding prostate cancer very early in the disease, perhaps too good. Problem is, this cancer doesn't play by the usual rules. Find it early, destroy it, save a life. That's how it's *supposed* to work, right?

But it's not that straightforward with prostate cancer. It's hard to determine the ideal strategy for screening, and it's not always clear what to do with it once we find the darn thing.

A man's checkup has long included an annual rectal exam of the prostate gland. In recent years, a blood test for the level of prostate-specific antigen (PSA), moved from obscurity into widespread use. We know for sure that PSA testing allows us to find prostate cancer *more often* and *at an earlier stage* than rectal exam alone. We also know that without screening, just waiting until symptoms develop often means it's time for the patient to get his affairs in order.

Yet, plenty of smart people question the value of routine PSA testing at all. They claim that overall patient health and the death rate from prostate cancer have not been clearly shown to improve with the widespread use of this sensitive blood test. They have a point.

How can we make sense of the conflicting information about prostate screening and then choose the best course of action when a *potential* problem is found? The answers, like the devil, are in the details, and there are a lot of details to consider.

First, here are some relevant facts and a little history. The prostate gland is one of the male sex glands. It lies right at the base of the urinary bladder, just in front of the rectum. This convenient location is why doctors always seem to be chasing you guys with gloves and a tube of lubricant. The gland can be easily examined by feeling it through the inner wall of the rectum. This reveals its size and shape and sometimes a cancer growing inside it.

But the convenient location doesn't necessarily draw customers. One reason thousands still die from prostate cancer is the very idea of the doc sticking a gloved finger up the butt. They postpone even thinking about it, never mind submitting to it. Understandable. Too often, fatal.

Because of this, the objectionable rectal exam may do more harm than good. One painful or emotionally traumatic exam may cause a patient to forget about regular checkups and miss other important screening exams as well.

Yes, this is far from a perfect screening method. The patient may be lucky enough to have a very small cancer that just happens to be growing in the back (posterior) lobe of the gland, which is the only area that can be felt through the rectal wall. Even then, a tumor big enough to be felt typically has been growing for some time and may have already reached an aggressive stage.

About twenty years ago, an obscure blood test, until then used only to watch for *recurrent* prostate cancer after its initial treatment, hit the screening scene. PSA testing promised deliverance for all us fanny-phobic males. Now you could tell your doctor where he *couldn't* shove it. With a simple blood test, physicians could identify early prostate cancer in the majority of patients.

I was filling in for a colleague when PSA tests were just getting introduced as a screening tool. My first experience with it came when I received results for two of his recently tested patients. Both had abnormally high levels of PSA. Not sure what that meant, I called a urologist buddy who suggested he see the patients. Both were in their 50's. Both had *normal* prostate rectal exams. Both had cancer. At that point, I was an instant believer in PSA screening.

About six months later, I received a call from a colleague and fellow internist. He told me he was one of the officers in a newly formed Independent Physician Association or IPA. These are medical groups responsible for managing insurance funds profitably for its members. We'd always been on the best of terms, but his group viewed my new habit of PSA testing as going beyond the accepted standard of care. As you may recall, many physicians prefer to play it safe and frown on colleagues who go above and beyond the *status quo* of the day. Especially when they have the added responsibility of managing costs to ensure profits.

PSA testing was considered expensive, and I was told, in no uncertain terms, to stop ordering them. I declined the offer. We agreed to disagree, but I had to inform patients they were responsible for the cost of the PSA test.

Then, in 1994, General H. Norman Schwarzkopf, having been recently diagnosed with prostate cancer, applied his celebrity as a Gulf War hero to raise consciousness about the importance of PSA testing. About the same time, the Wall Street legend, Mike Milken, just released from prison at the young age of 46, asked for a PSA test. His doctor told him he was too young, but Milken insisted. The result showed his PSA level was six times higher than normal. Soon after, Mr. Milken was diagnosed with *terminal* prostate cancer. The visibility of his diagnosis contributed to advancing PSA testing toward acceptance as the standard of care.

His bad news was to be good news for cancer patients. Mr. Milken, still very much alive as I write these words, had a long history of fascination with innovative approaches to treating cancer, yet was uninformed about the one that was attacking him. That didn't last long. Milken applied his influence and considerable fortune to advancing the diagnosis and treatment of prostate cancer, founding the Prostate Cancer Foundation, www.prostatecancerfoundation.org.

Prostate cancer was not considered a subject of polite conversation, of any kind of conversation, for that matter. But high profile patients like Schwarzkopf and Milken brought the issue out of the closet and increased public awareness. No surprise that increased awareness led to increased demand. Suddenly hundreds of thousands of PSA tests were conducted. No more threatening phone calls either, as most insurance carriers began to pay for PSA screening, no questions asked. A childish part of me would have liked to say, "I told you so," but I couldn't. Even after decades of use, the *overall* benefits of all this testing remains unclear.

A few final facts: The risk of both developing and dying from prostate cancer is almost two times higher for African-American men than for Caucasians and a bit lower for Asians. If you have a first-degree relative with prostate cancer, your risk more than doubles.

Last, and most importantly, 2 percent of men between 40 and 59 years of age are diagnosed with the disease, while 13 percent of men between 60 and 79 years of age are diagnosed with the disease. Age matters. Any man over age 85 has a *huge* likelihood of harboring prostate cancer, more than 75 percent. Yet stroke, heart disease, a different type of cancer, or accidents are much more likely to claim lives of prostate cancer patients in this age group.

Here's the thing. Prostate cancer is actually a pretty low-grade cancer, but it's so darn common that the 13 percent of patients who die from their disease add up to a very large death toll. In fact, if we never treated a single prostate cancer in America, more prostate cancer patients would die *with* their disease than *of* it.

The number of men diagnosed with prostate cancer has accelerated like a rocket in the past decade, from 165,000 new cases in 1994 to 235,000 new cases in 2005. This is not because the rate of prostate cancer is increasing but because it is being discovered in more patients with a sensitive test that is now widely used. In the past, statistically speaking, the majority of men with prostate cancer went to their graves for various other reasons, never knowing they had it.

If ignorance is bliss, PSA testing may be depriving a lot of men from blissful living. I say "so what?" *if* we are in fact saving lives. We're doing something right, because the death rate from prostate cancer in the U.S. has been dropping steadily, from 35,000 in 1994 to 30,000 in 2005. But does PSA screening get the credit?

I'd like to think so, since I've discovered dozens of prostate cancers in young men, 50 to 65 years old, and none of them has died from the disease to date. Yet in other countries, where PSA screening is less common, the death rate is also falling. Maybe some of my patients underwent invasive surgery or radiation treatments for a disease that might never have killed them in the first place.

The bottom line is prostate cancer doesn't play fair. We've become enormously effective at discovering it early. That's supposed to give us the upper hand! If it was a high-grade malignancy, like lung cancer, we could expect each and every case to behave aggressively, so early detection would translate clearly into lives saved.

As we'll see, when our PSA misbehaves, it can be from several different causes. The only way to know if the cause of a persistently-elevated PSA is cancer is with an invasive biopsy of the gland, which is not pleasant and comes with the risks of infection and other damage.

Even if we find cancer, it may not be aggressive, and for some patients it could be better to simply wait and watch. We do get *some* idea of how aggressive the tumor is by looking at the types of cells in the biopsy (see the Gleason Score in Appendix 11), but we don't always know the most important fact: whether or not the tumor has spread through the outer wall of the prostate gland. This is our best indicator of the need for aggressive treatment. But this information may not be discoverable until after the prostate gland is surgically removed.

Surgery is obviously even more unpleasant and comes with its own potential problems like urinary incontinence, impotence, even death from the procedure.

If we could prove that the falling death rate is directly related to the level of screening, then all the PSA tests, the biopsies, surgeries, and radiation treatments would be worth it. But it will take several more years before some well-designed studies resolve much of the uncertainty about this frustrating disease.

So what's a man to do? I can think of no other disease where our ability for early detection has come so far while our ability to prove its value in saving lives remains so elusive.

Here are some of the questions each man and his family must consider:

▶ **Should you get screened in the first place?**

▶ **If you do and the test raises concerns, under what circumstances should you have a biopsy?**

▶ **If a biopsy reveals cancer, what, if anything, should you do about it?**

I tend to believe that PSA testing, managed carefully, is a wise move for men expected to live another ten years or more. Screening after age 75, on the other hand, may be of little value from a *statistical* standpoint. That's not to say you won't die from the disease if you're older; in fact, over 90 percent of victims who die are over 65 years old. But screening gives us a ten-year head start on most prostate tumors, and if you find it in its early stages at age 75, it's unlikely that the cancer will become life-threatening for another ten years. Many men will die from other causes between ages 75 and 85. So screening after age 75 becomes a very personal choice.

At 75, a man in very good health might want to be just as aggressive in treating the disease as a 50-year-old. A man in heart failure or ravaged by other chronic disease, who isn't a good candidate for surgery, maybe shouldn't bother. Again, it's a personal choice. I offer screening to all my male patients over age 40 and actively encourage it up to age 75.

Before PSA screening is ordered, it's important for each man to know in advance what will happen, depending on all the possible results. Cancer can trigger such an emotional reaction that many patients feel a high PSA means somebody better cut that damned gland out yesterday! They need education before having the test, and may not be good candidates for screening if they aren't able to deal with the uncertainty that is sometimes necessary for wise management of abnormal test results.

About PSA

What results can you expect from a PSA test? Twenty years ago, if the result indicated prostate-specific antigen was below 4.0 nanograms per milliliter of blood, the test was considered normal, and anything above that was considered abnormal. This level was arbitrarily set so that a score of 4 ng/mL meant about a 25 percent chance of cancer. As you might suspect, this turned out to be oversimplified.

Back in the late 1980s, I screened a young man, Jay, whose PSA level was 1.4. The next year, it rose to 3.1, still below the level considered "normal." When it hit 5.3, two years after his first test, he was referred for biopsy, which found cancer. Jay had surgery to remove his prostate gland.

A few years after his surgery, Jay confronted me with the fact that an upward trend was obvious after his first two tests, and a recent article he found suggested I should not have waited a full year before his third test.

Thank goodness he's still with us. The only thing I could tell him was that at the time of his first two tests some considered me a renegade for even ordering the tests. Only a few years later, PSA *trending* became the state of the art.

PSA levels change. They go up slowly with age, they go up more quickly with cancer, or they can skyrocket overnight if the prostate becomes infected. In the first two cases, however, they only go one way – up. When the cause is infection, high PSA levels fall back to normal after successful treatment.

If you have PSA testing and the results are normal, it's important to do the test again every year. The absolute level of a single test is only part of the story; the *rate* of any increase, even if the scores are within the normal range, is just as important.

If the level starts out high or jumps up quickly over time, it's important to look further. A rectal exam should be part of every man's annual physical after age 50, and should also be done whenever there's an abnormal PSA result.

Evaluating for inflammation (prostatitis), and even treating for the condition when in doubt, may be reasonable before determining if a biopsy is necessary. Successful treatment for infection should lower the PSA level back to the pre-infection level.

If a moderately-high PSA level persists, between 4.0 and 10.0, and the prostate exam is normal, it's possible to look more closely at the situation with additional blood testing such as the *Percent Free* PSA which can give a better prediction of whether the high levels are from cancer or from the benign chronic enlargement that occurs in many men over the years. New studies are looking at certain antibodies, made by most men in response to prostate cancer, to determine if they are better predictors of cancer than PSA testing.

So at what point is a biopsy the smart move? I'm afraid there are no hard and fast guidelines that can be applied to all patients.

I would first rule out a prostate infection and then consider strongly recommending a biopsy in any of these situations:

▶ **the PSA is quite high (over 10 ng/mL)**

▶ **the PSA levels were rising quickly in a series of tests**

▶ **the physical exam reveals a 'lump'**

▶ **if secondary tests, such as percent free PSA, confirmed the likelihood of cancer.**

Patients with existing high-risk factors—African-American men and men with a family history of the disease, might have a somewhat lower threshold for going forward with the biopsy.

A biopsy will either reveal cancer cells or it won't. If there's evidence of cancer, it will either be of high or low grade, based on its Gleason Score. Prostate cancer is so common, and often of such a low grade, that if we took a biopsy from a 55-year-old Caucasian man with a *normal* rectal exam, *normal* PSA, and *no* family history of the disease, there would still be a 30 percent chance of finding cancer cells!

Fortunately, the chance of a *high-grade*, more aggressive cancer is less than 4 percent.

A biopsy isn't perfect, by the way. It doesn't sample every part of the gland and, even with ultrasound guidance to determine where to insert the biopsy needle, it's possible to miss a tumor. A biopsy can provide clear evidence of cancer, but if it does not find cancer, there's no guarantee it isn't there. More uncertainty.

Here is where a skilled urologist is important. All the factors unique to the patient must be considered by an expert in prostate cancer. They are the best guides in terms of a "wait and watch" approach, surgery, radiation, cryotherapy, or hormone therapy.

Sometimes the price of screening is living with uncertainty. I believe the ability to find and track small, unpredictable tumors, prostate and otherwise, will continue to improve with time and technology. In the process, we need to deal with our cultural terror of all-things-cancer. Current knowledge puts us so far ahead of where we were just twenty years ago, and this knowledge is allowing physicians to manage certain cases where the cancer can be kept on a short leash until it misbehaves enough to take more radical steps.

*"After applauding breast cancer awareness in this country,
I was astonished to discover that many people,
including healthcare providers, are unaware of the
most aggressive of all breast tumors."*

Chapter 20

Beyond the Mammogram

Breast cancer is scary, dangerous and common. With about 210,000 new cases every year, it ranks second only to lung cancer in killing women, over 40,000 deaths each year. It even beats lung cancer in killing younger women, those between 39 and 54. Unlike prostate cancer, every one of those 210,000 new tumors can be expected to behave very badly, very quickly if ignored.

Breast cancer has a disturbing way of being politically incorrect. With lung cancer, people often point to smoking as the cause, blaming victims for their self-destructive behavior. Smoking also encourages bladder and esophageal cancer. If we want to point fingers, we can also note that early sexual activity and multiple sexual partners clearly leads to more cervical cancer.

This is not so with breast cancer. It gleefully attacks *any* woman without rhyme or reason. And 1 percent of cases are actually in men. It's an equal opportunity invader. Women do not get a free pass by being chaste, beautiful, wealthy, young, perfect mothers, or health junkies. It strikes one in eight women, about 12.5 percent. It may not spread quite as fast as lung cancer, but it is no tortoise either. That's why mammograms need to be done *every* year, not once a decade like colonoscopy.

The good news is that breast cancer has reached top-of-the-mind awareness in our social consciousness. Pink ribbons and fund-raising invitations cross my path in one form or another every week. This high level of social consciousness is precisely why, for many victims, breast cancer would be a stupid reason for dying.

Sadly, impoverished or embattled women still tend to place breast screening low on the list of daily struggles, but for most American women, the *external* obstacles to breast education and screening have been removed.

Most readers know what they need to do in terms of yearly mammograms and self (or spousal) examination. For a quick refresher, screening guidelines and other breast cancer information are provided in Appendix 6. What I want to address here are the three side issues of breast cancer that have been in the media recently and may be misunderstood.

Estrogen Use and Breast Cancer

The media didn't waste a nanosecond reporting data linking combined estrogen-progesterone replacement therapy with increased risk for breast cancer, which was from the publication of a large prospective study known as the Women's Health Initiative. This well-done study left us our one existing triumph: that combination estrogen/progesterone therapy decreases the rate of uterine cancer. However, uterine cancer is a minor-league killer compared to heart disease and breast cancer. The study then dashed our hopes that hormone replacement could saves lives by reducing heart attack rates. It doesn't.

We hoped that research would reveal that combination estrogen/ progesterone therapy would lower breast cancer rates as it does with uterine cancer. It doesn't. It makes things worse. With a very dangerous disease that attacks one in eight women, the details of these findings matter a heck of a lot.

Yes, estrogen plus progesterone replacement therapy increases breast cancer risk. Now for the details. The *highest* estimates run about 20 percent greater risk, raising the average existing risk from 12.5 percent to about 15 percent. Obviously, this is not a good thing. Here's the problem. The important question, one that is rarely asked by people making critical, health-related decisions is this: "What are the risks of *not* taking hormone replacement after menopause?"

Until recently, that risk was considerable. Menopause leads to thinning bones (osteoporosis), which lead to fractures. Broken hips and spinal compression fractures continue to be a very common cause of death and disability in older women. One in four women will have a major fracture due to osteoporosis, which will lead to the death of one in four of these victims. Any reader who's dealt with these injuries themselves or in a family member knows what I'm talking about. Hormone replacement has been a major player in preventing the fractures that disable and ultimately claim lives.

Fortunately, new alternatives to estrogen replacement help re-grow bone, and some even reduce breast cancer risk at the same time.

So why would any woman take estrogen? The answer is simple, individual, and personal. Some women simply feel and function significantly better on hormone replacement after menopause or a total hysterectomy. Estrogen prevents hot flashes and excessive sweating, and it improves atrophied vaginal tissue for proper responsiveness in sexual functioning. Much less open to objective study are the benefits in concentration, mood, memory, libido, headache suppression, and the overall sense of well-being experienced in a subset of patients.

So what are your best estrogen "rules of engagement"? Consider the following points when you discuss this with your doctor.

▶ *Not* taking estrogen does *not* protect you from breast cancer. Your risk goes from 15 percent down to 12.5 percent. So what? Both are huge risks that make mammograms, self-examination, and a healthy dose of "breast cancer paranoia," the best defense for all women.

▶ The increased risk revealed by the Women's Health Initiative study is based on the combination of estrogen and progesterone therapy, *not* on estrogen alone. That part of the study did *not* show any increased risk for breast cancer.

▶ Estrogen is *not* the only way to prevent osteoporosis. There are great alternatives that are just as effective and possibly safer. One of these, Evista, has been proven to actually decrease breast cancer risk by up to 80 percent.

▶ Estrogen does *not* appear to help prevent heart disease as once hoped. Do not use it for that purpose.

▶ There is significant risk to taking estrogen therapy *of any kind* if you smoke or have a history of blood clots.

▶ Topical estrogen can be *very* effective in treating vaginal dryness and limits the amount of the hormone absorbed by the body in general, and, specifically, by breast tissue.

▶ Last, but very important: if you know in your heart that your mental, emotional, sexual, and/or physical life is richer when you take estrogen, don't throw the baby out with the bathwater. Tell your doctor what the benefits are for you personally. The increased risk of breast cancer or other dangers is small and, for some women, the loss of estrogen at menopause can be physically and emotionally devastating. The benefits of estrogen replacement are likely to be far greater for this group of women than for the population at large.

Remember, everything in life is a risk—what we do and what we don't do. It's difficult to measure the potential consequences of loss of estrogen like poor memory, mood disorders, and disrupted sexual relationships. Yet, they must not be ignored as often happens in the aftermath of media coverage that sensationalizes research findings without providing a true perspective of the benefits as well as the risks that physicians and patients must consider.

If life is better for an individual using hormone replacement, she should work closely with her healthcare provider to screen for breast cancer and any other concerns related to the therapy. In the real world, the "slightly nervous" use of hormone replacement often leads to greater diligence in screening, which means fewer breast cancers slip through the cracks.

I believe that this healthy paranoia is a life-saving benefit that can outweigh the slight increased risk that comes with combined hormone therapy.

Now that we're appropriately paranoid, is searching for lumps and annual mammograms really the best we can do? Other imaging machines exist for evaluating breast cancer, specifically MRI (magnetic resonance imaging) and PET (positron emission tomography.)

Is Mammogram the Best We've Got?

We've relied on mammograms for decades to find breast cancers as early as possible. And early matters. Small tumors, found early, are usually curable. Big tumors, found late, are deadly. While far from perfect, mammography has served us well and will continue to do so for some time. However, there are alternatives.

Recently, an excellent study from Holland looked at the usefulness of MRI scanning compared to either mammography or simple physical examination of the breasts. It studied women considered to be at *high risk* for breast cancer, either because they had a strong family history of breast cancer or a known genetic trait that increases risk.

In these women, invasive breast cancer was correctly diagnosed more often with MRI. The statistics are a bit confusing, but you can look at them more closely in Appendix 7.

Here are the highlights. The study looked at 1,909 women who received both an annual MRI *and* an annual mammogram, plus a breast examination every six months. Forty-five patients developed breast cancer during the course of the study. MRI scanning identified 32 of these and missed 13, while mammography found only 18, missing 27 cases! The MRI found more cancers—71 percent compared to only 40 percent for mammography, and a dismal 18 percent for physical examination of the breasts. This means MRI had a higher level of sensitivity for finding cancers that are actually there.

Now, remember specificity? It was lower for MRI than mammography, meaning that an MRI test is more likely to indicate there *is* cancer when in fact there *is not*. This required repeat imaging and breast biopsies that were negative for cancer.

The highest specificity was actually with physical examination of the breasts alone. But this only means that by the time physicians can feel something that appears to be cancer, it almost certainly is.

The difference in *specificity* between mammography and MRI was small, while the difference in *sensitivity* was huge. This is important, so stay with me. When these two qualities are combined, the MRI was clearly better.

Equally important, the tumors found in this study group of carefully screened women were smaller and involved fewer lymph nodes than tumors found in a matched group of women who received Holland's standard-of-care screening.

Does that mean mammography should be universally replaced by MRI scans? It's easy to draw that conclusion from the Holland study, which suggests the mammograms were nearly worthless. After all, they only found one-third of the cancers which, thankfully, were revealed by an MRI. However, there are a few important considerations about this study we must keep in mind.

First this was a study of women with *high risk factors*. Some so high, they had more than an 80 percent chance of developing breast cancer compared to average women with a 12.5 percent risk.

The focus of the research was to intercept high-risk women for screening *in anticipation* of cancer, so many of these patients were very young, in their 20s and 30s.

Radiologists will tell you that younger women have denser breast tissue, which is much harder to assess with a mammogram. MRI doesn't have the same problem with dense breast tissue. This factor accounted for many of the failures of mammography in the study.

In an average population, mammography accuracy is 88 percent compared to 40 percent in the study. The study also found that a mammogram was *superior* to MRI in detecting a specific type of breast cancer, ductal carcinoma in situ. So the question is not should MRI replace mammography, but does it make sense to use both MRI and mammogram to detect more cancers early.

The downside of this approach is the issue of false positives. MRI is more likely than mammography to indicate the possibility cancer is present when, in fact, there isn't one. This can lead to unnecessary:

▶ **additional imaging studies**
▶ **invasive biopsies**
▶ **anxiety**
▶ **higher costs**

So let's look closer at these "unnecessary" consequences of MRI scanning. The additional imaging is mostly harmless. There is a small radiation risk with extra mammograms but none with MRI. Breast MRI does involve the injection of a contrast agent, gadolinium, so an IV line must be placed, and there is a *very* tiny chance of a reaction to the gadolinium.

Unnecessary biopsies are another matter. Anyone contemplating MRI of the breast should know that a false-positive result is more likely than with mammogram alone. Rushing to perform a biopsy based on an "uncertain" finding comes with surgical risks. And rushing in is what happens. Unlike prostate cancer, where we don't yet know if early, frequent biopsies actually save lives, we know that aggressive biopsy of breast abnormalities often does.

It's not as though breast biopsy isn't already an epidemic! A mammogram is good at finding "abnormalities" in the breast but can't differentiate between malignant and non-malignant abnormalities, which makes a biopsy the rule, not the exception.

As for anxiety, once again, we see the need for a well thought out plan of how the results will be handled *before* deciding to use MRI for breast screening. If you plan to peek under a lot of rocks when screening your body for cancer, you need to be prepared for what you find. In many cases, what we find raises more questions. And, it may take several months of uncertainty before you get the answers.

Then, as always, there's the cost issue. MRI is still very expensive, about 10 times the cost of a mammogram. Many professionals who oppose certain current screening policies assume the policy is based on concern about widespread insurance coverage. To increase breast cancer screening costs by tenfold in this country would have a huge impact on the insurance industry.

On the other hand, if a test makes good medical sense for a particular patient, it does so regardless of who pays for it. For newer tests, it is most likely going to be the patient.

Who should get MRI breast screening in addition to mammography? A cavalier answer would be: Any well-informed woman who wants it and is willing to pay for it and accept the possibility of finding something too small or atypical to offer definitive results. Not knowing is not easy. It often means additional testing and a period of living with uncertainty.

Having said that, I encourage women at *high risk* for breast cancer to consider an MRI as well as a mammogram. There is clearly a better chance for early detection in this group, and I believe the benefits outweigh the additional cost and the potential for false-positive results. This is especially true for young, high-risk women more likely to have dense breasts or who have breast implants that can diminish the sensitivity of mammography.

Are *You* At High Risk?

Some people are born at high risk for breast cancer. Anyone who carries genes such as BRCA1 or BRCA2 should consider himself or herself at high risk. These genes are sometimes found in families with multiple cases of breast or ovarian cancer. The need for genetic testing is a discussion for your physician or a genetics counselor.

Typically, physicians use the GAIL questionnaire, which helps to determine a person's 5-year risk of breast cancer. It's based on the following information:

▶ *Age*

▶ *Age at menarche (onset of menstruation)*

▶ *Age at your first child's (live) birth*

▶ *Number of first-degree relatives (mother, sister[s], and/or daughter[s]) with breast cancer)*

▶ *Number of previous breast biopsies (whether positive or negative)*

▶ *At least one biopsy with atypical hyperplasia (overly exuberant tissue growth)*

You can calculate risk with a computer program available online. One location is: http://bcra.nci.nih.gov/brc/start.htm.

However, the limitation, as with other common risk-assessment tools, is that the GAIL score is indirect and statistical in nature, designed to predict risk in a population of women. It cannot respond to you, a unique individual, who didn't come from a conveyer belt.

It also relies, to some degree, on the person being a mother and actually having a fair number of relatives. What do you do if you're from a small or dispersed family or one that keeps its medical secrets? What do you do if you're adopted? The point here, ladies: a low risk based on the GAIL score is *not* a substitute for a mammogram and self-examination. And, if breast cancer runs heavily in your family, consider the MRI.

Just a few words about Pet Scans. Positron emission tomography is a promising technology for very early detection of breast and other cancers. (Discussed briefly in Appendix 8.) They are already being used to detect the spread of known breast cancer throughout the body.

It relies on the metabolism of the cancer itself to actively absorb mildly radioactive food. This causes a tumor to "glow in the dark" to the eyes of the scanner. Current obstacles to widespread use include cost, about $3,000, limited availability of the radioactive tracer, which must be made fresh in an "on-site" cyclotron just before use, and limitations on how detailed an image will be with current scanners that are mostly designed to look at the whole body.

Yet progress is being made on the development of smaller scanners that only surround the breast, allowing better resolution of small tumors and at much lower cost for the equipment. Also, radioactive isotope distribution centers are becoming more widespread. As the volume of Pet Scanning increases for its many other uses, this will make transportation and availability of this short-lived product much greater.

For now, get a mammogram without fail every single year of your life from age 40 on. If you have a strong family history of breast cancer or have had genetic testing that places you at high risk, and especially if you have dense breast tissue or implants that can complicate things, talk with your healthcare provider about the need for an MRI screening.

The good news is that our ability to save lives in breast cancer is slowly improving. Stay tuned for new developments in our quest to find and cure *all* breast cancers. It's up to you to stay abreast (sorry) of the issues, so you don't miss important opportunities, like MRI for high-risk women.

Finally, a warning about a unique breast cancer killer.

Inflammatory Breast Cancer

After applauding breast cancer awareness in this country, I was astonished to discover that many people, including healthcare providers, are unaware of the most aggressive of all breast tumors. Perhaps that's because it is, thankfully, so rare. Only about 3 percent of breast cancers fall in this category, but it grows faster and in a different manner than most breast tumors.

We usually expect to find the dreaded "lump" in an otherwise soft breast. Not so with inflammatory breast cancer, IBC. It grows in sheets of cells that form small separate "nests," often just below the skin, not as deep as the usual suspects. The tumor cells block the normal lymphatic drainage of the tissue causing the surface of the breast to become inflamed, which typically presents as warm skin with color changes.

Initial symptoms of IBC come on quickly and include any of the following:

▶ **a rapid, unusual increase in the size of one breast (up to a full cup size bigger)**

▶ **nipple discharge**

▶ **increased skin temperature**

▶ **a change in the nipple itself such as inversion, dimpling or retraction**

▶ **skin changes, such as a blotchy red rash**

▶ **itching of the breast or nipple**

▶ **a lump or thickening of breast tissue**

▶ ***any* lymph node swelling under the arm or around the collar bone**

▶ **and, contrary to the common belief that breast cancer doesn't initially hurt, IBC frequently causes pain or soreness in the breast.**

Mammograms usually miss early inflammatory breast cancer, because it doesn't form lumps early on. And, the symptoms are misleading. They're similar to a breast infection known as mastitis, and doctors often prescribe antibiotics in error. If a response to antibiotics for a breast infection is not evident after a week, a biopsy should be performed or a referral made to a breast specialist immediately.

IBC also strikes women an average of ten years younger than other breast cancers, often pregnant or nursing mothers. The few cases I've seen have been in African-American women in their 20s, sadly, a particularly at-risk group. Even teenage girls develop the disease and may be too embarrassed to talk about symptoms with a parent or physician, wasting the precious time they may need to survive.

Yes, early *really* matters with IBC because it is so fast-growing. Since the lymph channels are already involved at the initial diagnosis, it is considered at stage 3 level of cancer spread. The scale only goes to stage 4. *Immediate* recognition and treatment are the only chance for a cure. Although it is a rare form of breast cancer, all women need to know the symptoms, because it's impossible to predict who it will strike. It is not a disease that can wait for an annual doctor visit and mammogram.

Which brings me to the last point in this chapter:

Woman, Know Thy Own Breasts

Your breasts are not like any others in the world. They are unique in size, shape, texture, density, and vulnerability to cancer. They are also inherently lumpy and irregular on the inside. No one, including your doctor, can know your breasts as well as you do. You've lived with them longer and recognize how they've changed over the years. That means you are the expert, the one person most likely to detect a lump, bump, dimple, or discharge that needs to be evaluated. Providing, of course, you are paying attention.

I wrote this book in part to *decrease* the general fear about cancer by telling you about state-of-the-art technology for early detection and treatment.

Breast cancer is the exception to this rule. Please, BE PARANOID. Be vigilant about self-examination of your breasts, and make sure all the females over 12 years of age in your home talk openly and freely about self-exams. And guys, if you are shy about the subject, get over it. They're only breasts, and they're not worth dying for.

I can only tell you that in my professional experience, I have never *ever* regretted promoting the policy of "assuming the worst" when it comes to breast cancer. Bad things happen to the greatest women.

"Our last two killers are not related to cancer, heart disease, or infection. One likes women, the other prefers men."

Chapter 21
Finishing Off Some Killers

Welcome to the home stretch. We've covered the high-volume cancer killers. Now let's touch on some less common but equally lethal tumors and a few non-malignant threats.

Unfortunately, for some forms of cancer there is nothing useful to be shared about prevention or screening. Diseases like pancreatic cancer or malignant brain tumors just materialize and kill. Some cancer battles can only be fought, often unsuccessfully, after the disease has declared itself and already has an upper hand.

Someday we may have the sophisticated technology for whole-body cancer detection and cures for currently hopeless tumors. We aren't there yet. Worrying in advance about such things makes no sense. You'll either get them, unlikely, or you won't. We have no control at all, and chronic worry itself will create other health problems.

But the other cancers we'll review here deserve your attention, because they can be found early. In some cases, it is not yet clear if aggressive screening makes a difference in survival. This is *not* the case, however, with the beauty mark from hell.

Malignant Melanoma

Malignant melanoma uses a killing strategy just the opposite of the colon cancer tortoise. This cancer hits the ground running and moves like a locomotive. Colon cancer requires us to thread fancy cameras into unwelcoming places to find it. Melanoma hides in plain sight.

It is a cancer of pigment-producing cells found mostly in the skin, but also in the eyes, ears, and even in our gut and brain. To call it a skin cancer is not exactly accurate, because its cells are actually of nerve origin. But the skin and other visible areas of our bodies are the only locations where we are likely to identify these tumors in time to stop them. Fortunately, the skin is also the most likely crime scene.

Unlike other skin cancers, melanoma doesn't rely on accumulated sun exposure to set it off. It can occur where the sun never shines. If malignant melanoma was *simply* a sun cancer, we would expect it to be mainly on the face and hands, the areas most exposed to the sun. Indeed, another much more common but far less dangerous skin cancer, basal cell carcinoma, is found almost exclusively in these areas.

For reasons unknown, melanoma seems to favor the back and legs. I've also found these lesions on the bottom of the feet and other parts of the body normally covered at least by a bathing suit.

There is, however, a direct link between high sun exposure in childhood and malignant melanoma later in life. The incidence of this cancer is increasing steadily in America, but even more so in Australia and New Zealand where ozone depletion has opened the sky to more ultraviolet radiation.

The attack rate of melanoma in these countries is almost four times higher than in the U.S. So sun does matter. Do not let your children sunburn. At the same time, shade dwellers get it, too. One theory is that more infrequently exposed skin suffers more damage when it gets an "occasional burn," which could explain melanoma's favorite sites and its blessedly higher prevalence on the skin than in hidden, internal tissues.

Malignant melanoma can occur at *any* age, from early childhood to late in a long life. It favors Caucasians, especially men. And, while it represents only 4 percent of U.S. skin cancers, it's responsible for the vast majority of skin cancer deaths, close to 8,000 in 2005. We record almost 60,000 new cases each year, so the good news is that the cure rate is pretty solid in America—about 91 percent. And the cure rate continues to rise because of early detection, more awareness of a mole's danger signs, and less sunburn in the younger generations. The one group that lags behind in survival are middle-age and older white men.

The qualities known to raise a person's risk are:

▶ **a fair complexion, excessive childhood sun exposure (especially blistering childhood sunburns)**

▶ **an increased number of common and dysplastic moles (known as Dysplastic Nevus Syndrome)**

▶ **a family history of melanoma**

▶ **male gender and older age.**

People at high risk, especially with Dysplastic Nevus Syndrome or a prior history of any skin cancer, should be under the ongoing surveillance of a dermatologist. Sometimes photographic studies of the skin can be employed to help detect new or changing moles against a busy background.

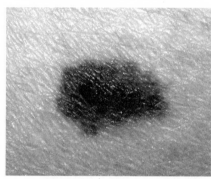

Know the melanoma. Its irregular shape, ragged borders and non-uniform color deserves immediate attention.

Malignant melanoma is most commonly characterized as a darkish brown or black lesion, initially flat. The lesions are more "seen" than "felt" at first. In many ways, they resemble an ink-blot where one side does not match the other. As they grow, they appear to spread *under* the surface of the skin. They are irregular in shape with notched or ragged borders. They can also be irregular in color, sometimes displaying shades of tan, brown, black, red or blue. (See the ABCDE criteria in Appendix 9.)

Most importantly, they grow and change. It can be possible to tell the difference in size in the course of just weeks in one of these lesions. Although they can arise in existing moles, at least 60 percent show up as new dark spots.

There are also variations from the common *Superficial Spreading Melanoma* described above.

Nodular Melanoma is also usually dark but not flat. It's raised and grows very fast, and it accounts for about 20 percent of all melanomas.

A really sneaky type, the Amelanotic Melanoma doesn't make the dark pigment we rely on for detection but is, thankfully, rare.

If caught early, melanoma is easy to remove, and the risk of spreading (metastases) and death is very remote. On the other hand, if allowed to grow unchecked, they quickly tunnel into deeper tissues, into the lymphatic system and from there, all over the body.

For this reason, *any* suspicious mole, flat or otherwise, that appears to have changed or appears to be new, or simply to have become more prominent or is developing less regular edges, should be evaluated by a physician at the earliest possible time.

I have referred several patients to dermatologists for lesions that did not seem to be all that abnormal, only to rejoice for being overly-cautious when the results were malignant melanoma.

Pay attention to your body. Check your skin all over on a regular basis. Have someone else check hard-to-see areas like your back. For couples, take literally the expression, "You watch my back, I'll watch yours."

Do not think your annual doctor's visit is enough. Malignant melanoma must be detected within months of its appearance for safe, complete removal. With a 91 percent cure rate, thanks to public awareness and proactive patients, neglecting a new, strange, fascinating beauty mark is another stupid reason for dying.

Esophageal Cancer

Here is another cancer that is not very common, but it does kill its victims. And the incidence of esophageal cancer is on the rise, increasing at an average rate of over 40 percent a decade.

There are many proposed reasons for this alarming trend. The most convincing ones point to acid reflux, which stems from factors such as obesity and hiatal hernias, problems generally on the rise. Other major risk factors include tobacco and excessive exposure to alcohol.

The most common approach to disease of the esophagus has been to wait for people to report symptoms of heartburn or reflux of stomach contents into the esophagus, gastroesophageal reflux disease or GERD, and then treat them with acid-reducing medications such as Zantac or Nexium.

More recently, we have been performing a procedure called endoscopy in patients with heartburn to visually examine the lining of the esophagus with a miniature scope. But what most people (and too many physicians) don't realize, is that about half of all people who are destined to develop cancer of the esophagus actually have *no* symptoms of heartburn or reflux until the opportunity for a cure has left the building.

In light of all this, there is medical debate whether people over 50, even those with no symptoms, should consider undergoing endoscopic screening of the esophagus every 4 to 5 years. As with colonoscopy, a camera on a hose is passed down the throat into the esophagus, stomach, and then upper intestine. I suppose you're not surprised that it's expensive. It's also somewhat invasive and requires intravenous sedation. All in all, you wouldn't consider it a good time.

The FDA recently approved a new technology, the PillCam®, for use in the U.S. As the name suggests, it is a camera the size of a large vitamin that's swallowed like a pill. As it travels down the esophagus, it rapidly flashes light, snapping 14 pictures per second, which are transmitted to a receiver outside the patient's body. The entire procedure takes a few minutes. The PillCam® exits in a bowel movement.

Since we don't know if the procedure leads to better survival from esophageal cancer, I recommend it *electively* to men and women over 50 who have *no significant symptoms* of heartburn or reflux, especially if they have been a smoker or heavy drinker or if they are obese.

I do not recommend it for patients *with* any symptoms of heartburn or reflux; they need endoscopy, the gold standard. Anyone who has had a normal endoscopy examination in the last 5 years is not likely to benefit from this test, and those who've had abnormal endoscopies should get *repeat* endoscopies.

It is important to realize that the PillCam® is only a screening tool, used to look for abnormal tissue in the esophagus. Any suspicious finding will require a followup endoscopy to biopsy the area. Like the EBT HeartScan, the PillCam® is not likely to be covered by insurance any time soon. Currently, the cost of the procedure runs between $1200 and $1500.

This is a very new field, and at least two things will surely change. The cost will drop over time, and the recommendations for who should and should not have this screening will become clearer. For now, your best bet is to stay away from tobacco and excessive drinking, and report any symptoms of heartburn or reflux to you physician.

Bladder Cancer

This cancer is more common than you may realize, responsible for about 50,000 new cases a year and 11,000 deaths.

Currently, the most we do to detect it is check urine samples once a year for blood that may not be visible to the naked eye. The experts with The United States Preventive Services Task Force (USPSTF) don't even recommend that much, since there is not yet evidence that it leads to saving lives.

Microscopic levels of blood in the urine are pretty common and usually don't mean cancer of the bladder (or kidney). Small amounts of blood can come from other things like bladder or prostate infection, kidney stones, toxic medications, heavy exercise, menstruation, sexual activity, and the list goes on. On top of that, urine screening can easily miss cancers that aren't bleeding on the day of our physical.

I once gave a clean bill of bladder-health to a patient and colleague based on a normal urine test. Six months later he was urinating blood. He had an aggressive bladder cancer not recognized by the urine test. You can bet I reviewed his chart to make sure we hadn't missed anything.

I'm happy to say he's fine now after taking decisive, aggressive action. Had he failed to notice the blood in his urine, his cancer could have spread like wildfire. If his annual physical six months earlier had been performed a day before or after, it's possible the urine test would have detected blood. It's a roll of the dice because these tumors bleed *intermittently*.

There is more we can do to identify bladder cancer beyond the basic urine test. Cytology testing requires submitting that same urine sample to an expert, a pathologist, who can detect both bladder and kidney cancer cells in urine samples. We know we can discover both bladder and kidney cancer earlier this way.

The catch is that while cancer cells in the urine clearly means there is a problem, the *absence* of cancer cells does not. A single annual cytology test can still miss some tumors. Since there's little downside to cytology screening (false-positive results are extremely rare), I currently offer it as part of an annual screening to my patients. I tell them what I just told you—the proof of a benefit from earlier detection doesn't exist yet. I also let them know they'll probably have to pay the $45 out-of-pocket cost.

On the horizon, there is excitement about a substance called *telomerase*, found in certain cancer cells, as a tool for detecting tumor cells in the urine. A chemical test of the urine for this protein is yielding some very promising results.

Ovarian Cancer

Cancer of the ovary made headlines when it deprived the world of two beloved comedic actresses, Gilda Radner and Madeline Kahn.

It's a relatively rare disease, attacking only 17 out of 100,000 women. But it makes up for this by its stealth and aggression, usually spreading beyond the ovary before it's discovered. It takes the life of over 16,000 American women each year.

A common blood test, CA-125, will mistakenly read high in 1 out of 50 women tested, yielding hundreds of false-positive results for every correct diagnosis.

Transvaginal ultrasound of the ovaries can help find the cancer earlier but, like the blood test, is not definitive; it will often see things that are questionable.

The ovaries are exasperating when it comes to capturing their image. They are naturally lumpy and irregular from the monthly gyrations of growing and reabsorbing egg follicles, as well as forming cysts of all shapes and sizes. This plagues the search for ovarian cancer with all the problems in screening discussed in Chapter 11. Uncertain results about such a scary cancer naturally creates anxiety and leads to more testing procedures, some of which are invasive.

Unlike the colon, the breast, and even the prostate, the ovaries are *not* in an easily accessed location. A biopsy is a big deal, requiring major surgery. So, for this fairly rare tumor, it must be considered that the risk of testing may outweigh the benefits.

Screening for ovarian cancer needs to improve. At this point, there are encouraging studies indicating that a group of 4 blood protein tests, taken together, demonstrate much greater sensitivity and specificity in identifying ovarian cancer. More time is needed to know if these tumor markers will consistently prove accurate and useful. In the meantime, we must make good selective use of the screening available.

Ovarian cancer runs in families. A single first-degree relative with ovarian cancer increases a woman's risk to five percent and two such relatives raises it to seven percent. Screening makes sense for these women. Even tests with a high false-positive rate start to become useful in a high-risk population.

As always, a well thought out plan between you and your doctor is needed *before* undertaking such screening to avoid "panic testing" followed by needless surgeries based on uncertain screening results.

The USPSTF recommends against routine screening for ovarian cancer.

However, with all the considerations mentioned, I do offer trans-vaginal ultrasound to patients but discourage CA-125 testing for women who do not have a family history of the disease. Real progress in ovarian cancer screening seems to be around the corner and will be closely followed on our website.

Testicular Cancer

Ready for a refreshing change? Here's a cancer where screening is *almost* superfluous. Made famous by cycling hero Lance Armstrong and his "live strong" yellow wrist bands, this rare tumor is now 95 percent curable. About 7,000 teens and young men get the disease annually, but less than 350 die as a result. Twenty-five years ago, the death rate was ten times higher. With modern chemotherapy, the cure rate of even widely metastasized tumors approaches 80 percent. Of course, we want a 100 percent cure rate, so the earlier the cancer is found the better.

Though it accounts for less than 1 percent of U.S. cancers, it ranks as the most common in this young male population. For unknown reasons, it's four times more common in white men than African Americans.

When discovered, testicular cancer may be anywhere from the size of a pea to the size of an egg. Most often, the patient finds the tumor himself either by careful self examination, yes, probably a rare event, or by noticing a symptom such as swelling, or occasional pain in a single testicle. Other findings include a full feeling or a fluid buildup in the scrotum. The patient might also have generalized symptoms such as fatigue, something that is not common in boys and men between 15 and 34 years of age.

On the other hand, there is a very long list of perfectly benign reasons for swelling in the scrotum. This is why any abnormal finding must be brought to the doctor's attention as soon as it's discovered to be further evaluated. This is often done with the aid of ultrasound.

Besides being male, Caucasian, and in the physical prime of life, the risk for testicular cancer goes up five to ten times if a brother or father had it or if the patient was born with an undescended testicle, even if it was repositioned with surgery. HIV infection may also raise the risk. The causes for this cancer are unknown, so there's no good advice on how to avoid it.

Advisors at the USPSTF do not recommend *any* routine screening, not even on the part of the physician at check-up. They don't encourage self-examination either. It's not that they don't care about the lives of young men. Their job is to identify and encourage only those screening practices that show evidence of saving lives. With the low incidence and high cure rates of this cancer in America, they are concerned about the harm of increasing anxiety and the cost of unnecessary testing.

Of course, *you* won't overreact, right? So self-exam is optional. I recommend it with the proviso that patients keep the *dangers of screening* in mind. We are likely to find many more masses that are not cancerous, and time is not the fierce enemy here that it can be with other types of cancer. Therefore, in most cases, watchful waiting makes the most sense.

The good news is that while early detection is preferable, this is a situation that doesn't scream for immediate intervention.

Cervical Cancer

Let's wrap up all this talk of cancer with some good news.

Our assault on cervical cancer during the last century is one of humanity's great victories over cancer. While today 3,700 American women do die each year from cervical cancer, in 1955 it was closer to 15,000.

Pap Smear testing is credited with cutting the death rate from this awful disease by 75 percent. And that number is about to get even better.

As with breast cancer, this is another area where a better-than-average adherence to common screening guidelines is paying off. Women know they should get checked, and most show up reluctantly for their regular exam. Unlike breast cancer, more like colon cancer, cervical cancer grows slowly in the beginning. It can be developing for years before it becomes incurable. So, even a few missed annual screenings are not likely to give this cancer free rein. *Please, do not take that as permission to skip your annual Pap Smear.* Cervical cancer screening guidelines, as of this writing, can be found in Appendix 10.

In addition to our ability to find cervical cancer increasing with every improved variation of the Pap Smear test, brilliant scientists have uncovered the cause of almost all cervical cancer, Human Papilloma Virus (HPV), and have just provided us with the first vaccine to protect women from this invisible, cancer-causing infection.

Merck, the pharmaceutical company so recently vilified for Vioxx, just released Gardasil, which involves a series of three injections a few months apart. Gardasil initially showed 100 percent protection against the cause(s) of cervical cancer. Other companies are slated to release similar HPV vaccines soon. Vaccination is currently recommended for girls and women between the ages of 9 and 26, preferably before onset of sexual activity.

As with all new state-of-the-art technology in medicine, we're faced with the same obstacles. Initially, not every insurance plan will jump to cover it. It costs about $360 for the whole series, so some women will refuse to foot the bill. Concern about as-yet-unknown side-effects will also delay it's use in some families and some doctor's offices. But in this case, there's the potential for another obstacle.

Some groups are gearing up to oppose vaccination, despite a survey showing that 80 percent of parents favor vaccinating their daughters. "Abstinence is the best way to prevent HPV," said a member of a leading Christian lobby group. The groups claim that giving the HPV vaccine to young women could be interpreted as a license to engage in premarital sex.

Arguments like the one above, even if they sound reasonable to some parents, simply make no sense. None. There is no evidence whatsoever that sexual activity in teenagers and young adults has anything at all to do with a knowledge of HPV. Half of all sexually-active women between 18 and 22 in the U.S. are already infected, which can cause cancer decades later. To bank on the fantasy that "your" child will never join that group but will only marry another virgin, is simply unrealistic about 95 percent of the time.

We have long been vaccinating our kids against Hepatitis B, a potentially lethal disease spread by sex and drug use. There is no evidence that this immunity encourages sexual activity or drug use.

By their logic, we should also ban condoms and other forms of birth control, things that certainly *do* relate to sexual activity. I cannot imagine a 15-year-old girl, getting vaccinated for a cancer she never heard of, thinking, "Oh wow! *Now* I can have sex!" Sadly, some groups that oppose life-saving advancements for fear they will encourage young people to become sexually active clearly do not understand how kids think or what leads them to make decisions that are not in their best interest.

Consider this: 80 percent of cervical cancer deaths occur in developing countries, where cultural and religious taboos will make the battle for acceptance of the vaccine harder than in the U.S. Young women become victims of their own cultures. While it's frustrating that time and lives will be wasted before the full benefits of this vaccine will be realized, it is one of a number of vaccines still being developed that have the potential to be among western medicine's greatest gifts to humanity.

What a pleasant thing to put the discussion of cancer behind us, at least for now. I'll ask you to bring it out of the closet only about once a year to refresh and update your own screening plans.

We've only considered here those cancers that are big-ticket killers, smaller killers but easy to detect, or which seem on the verge of new breakthroughs in screening that could save lives. But we didn't scratch the surface of cancer treatment. That would take a book on each specific type. My goal here has been to encourage you to take a role in finding cancer and other killers sooner rather than later, and to do so safely, rationally, and aggressively as an informed patient.

HIV

Once the kiss of death, now "treatable" in so many ways. And early treatment matters. It provides the best chance of halting the progression from HIV infection to the fatal AIDS syndrome.

My screening recommendations are no different here than those of the United States Preventive Services Task Force (USPSTF). We should look for this infection in those at high risk of having it, and treat aggressively when it's found.

Who's at high risk?

Men who have had sex with men, and all people with a background that includes one or more of the following:

▶ **intravenous drug use**

▶ **blood transfusion received between 1978 to 1985**

▶ **unprotected sex with multiple partners**

▶ **sex in exchange for money or drugs**

▶ **sex with someone who exchanged sex for money or drugs**

▶ **past or present sexual relations with HIV-positive partners or high-risk partners**

▶ **a history of other sexually transmitted diseases**

▶ **exposure to possible HIV contamination through direct needle stick or other accident in a high-risk setting**

Research also shows that people who request HIV testing, despite reporting none of these risk factors, are at increased risk for

HIV infection, probably because they have risk factors that they do not want to report.

The blood tests used to diagnose HIV infection are highly accurate. Early diagnosis increases the benefits of treatments that prevent opportunistic infections that complicate HIV. Close monitoring identifies the first signs that indicate treatment is needed. In pregnant women, early diagnosis allows treatment for preventing the spread of infection from mother to infant.

Those without any high-risk behaviors or experiences have a remarkably low chance of being infected.

Our last two killers are not related to cancer, heart disease, or infection. One likes women, the other prefers men. Neither comes with the sickening punch of a diagnosis of cancer, but they kill all the same. Both are also easier to treat.

Osteoporosis

Thin bones. Who dies from thin bones? Sadly, millions do. The risk of being dead within one year of a hip fracture is at least 20 percent! And there are over 700,000 hip fractures every year in this country. Do the math. This killer is right up there with the worst cancers.

The problems emerge like this: Fracture leads to falling, occasionally deadly. Repair of the break requires surgery, also dangerous in this older population. Reduced activity during recovery increases the chance for dangerous blood clots in the legs and pelvis that can break free and kill. An immobile patient is more isolated and vulnerable to depression, fear, anxiety, stress about finances, and whatever might be ahead, all guaranteed to shave time off their lifespan.

Osteoporosis is usually a disease of older people, and old people don't recover well from fractures and immobility. Any reader who has cared for an elderly person with a fracture knows what I'm talking about. Of all patients with hip fracture, about 20 percent require long-term nursing care, and 50 percent lose some or all of their ability to live independently.

Compression fractures of the vertebrae, common in osteoporosis, shorten a person's life expectancy not only because it places them into a statistical group where another major break is more likely, but also by causing intractable and immobilizing pain. Again, causing a general decline in health and deforming the chest and spine, which leads to lung and heart problems.

In many cases, a fall is not the cause of a broken hip; osteoporosis is the cause of the fall. The patient may believe she fell off the front step and broke her hip when, in fact, her hip fractured while walking, causing her to fall.

These are some very frail bones. Although we may notice a loved one is shrinking or stooped over, clear signs of osteoporosis, the problem in many people remains invisible. Too often, the first sign of osteoporosis is a fracture that shortens life and robs it of quality in the process.

Bones thin with age, especially in women after menopause. Bones remain very much alive and active throughout our entire lives, constantly remodeling themselves. There's an ongoing balancing act between two types of bone cells—those that reabsorb bone, and those that lay it down. When the balance is upset by conditions that slow the bone-growing cells *or* stimulate the bone reabsorbing cells, the result is osteoporosis.

Our bodies lay down increasing bone only during the first 30 years of life. Failure to do so during this 30-year opportunity can lead to lifelong osteoporosis as well. This is a serious problem in girls and young women who become overly thin and/or exercise excessively.

Our cultural obsessions with thinness and sports are life-threatening by themselves. The female ballet dancer or runner who stops menstruating because of weight loss or extreme exercise is actually destroying her body, and the destruction is permanent.

Estrogen in women and testosterone in men are important for more than sexual development. They ensure our bones keep up with growth. Since all women stop producing all but a tiny amount of estrogen after age 50 or so, it's no wonder sweet old ladies with broken hips are filling emergency rooms everywhere.

Many men also develop osteoporosis, and they do even worse than women at surviving their fractures. They're just as susceptible to the other diseases and medications that thin the bones. And it's now recognized that men gradually lose testosterone with age.

Half of all women and a quarter of all men over 50 will suffer an osteoporosis-related fracture in their lifetime. There are 44 million Americans, including 14 million men, with low bone mass (osteopenia), or the more severe osteoporosis. The difference is a matter of degree.

Overall, low bone density affects one in two adults. Many, if not most, don't know they have a problem, because despite all we know about osteoporosis, it continues to be under-evaluated and under-treated.

This is tragic, considering medical science now has a solid grip on treatment. Many new and established therapies can prevent and even reverse bone loss.

In the past, estrogen replacement has been used in older women as a strategy for slowing bone loss. That has declined in response to concern about estrogen's role as a risk factor for breast cancer and other problems with its use. Chapter 20 will refresh your memory. Fortunately, newer, more effective medications are now available, some of which have the added benefit of decreasing breast cancer risk up to 80 percent. Other agents go beyond just slowing bone loss and actually re-grow bone.

Can we prevent osteoporosis? Sure, to some degree. This is one of those situations where our traditional "use as little as possible," conservative approach to medication may be getting in our way. We react to osteoporosis, or it's milder form, osteopenia, only after the damage is done.

Prevention with adequate intake of calcium, 1200 to 1500 mg per day, and Vitamin D along with exercise to keep bone remodeling active, is widely taught.

In my experience, many women walk away with this information thinking calcium supplements and being active are enough. Yet, every new study that's come out shows that supplements and exercise are much more ineffective than originally thought. Calcium and Vitamin D are certainly important raw materials, but just as in building a home, raw materials aren't much use without blueprints, workers, and tools to put them into use. Osteoporosis is seldom a lack of building blocks; it's because the bone-growing machinery isn't adequately engaged.

Real prevention in the future will likely include the elective use of bone-sparing medications after menopause but *before* development of osteoporosis.

The medication raloxifene (Evista), is known to both prevent bone loss *and* breast cancer at the same time. In a perfect world, we would be able to predict which women will lose bone mineral density before it starts.

For now, the trick is to identify the person with the problem. There are plenty of clues that a patient may have thin bones: a history of fracture; loss of body height; diseases such as overactive thyroid or rheumatoid arthritis; lactose intolerance and celiac sprue; alcoholism; low blood levels of Vitamin D; and the use of certain drugs like prednisone, lithium, phenytoin, and some chemotherapy agents, to name just a few.

However, the smart approach, once again, is to know for sure by testing individuals. The risk of a fracture is most closely associated with the bone density itself. The best test for this is the bone DEXA scan (dual energy x-ray absorptiometry.) It's a painless fancy x-ray procedure that accurately measures bone density in several places, usually the hip, the spine and the arm. These results offer a baseline for comparison from one year to the next, which enables us to track bone loss and monitor the success or failure of treatment.

Who should get a DEXA? I recommend the first one for any woman beginning at 50, sooner if she is at higher risk for osteoporosis. Followup testing is spaced out according to the results of prior scans. Bone loss is typically a downward spiral, and intercepting and slowing it early makes a huge difference in the quality and length of one's life.

For men, I recommend it to those who demonstrate hypogonadism, low testosterone production, or who have other risk factors such as cortisone use or thyroid disease. I have recently begun recommending at least a one-time DEXA for all men at age 60 or older, and, as of this writing, Medicare is also considering paying for a one-time test in men. The cost is not high, a few hundred dollars, and the risks of the test are negligible – a tiny bit of radiation.

Despite the very real dangers of osteoporosis, the inherent fear of impending death does not plague the discovery of thin bones the way it does with cancer. This has made the management of bone density "bad news" easier. Doctors and patients don't get crazy with fear or an urge to overreact. When a problem is found, a few simple blood tests are needed to see if some untreated, underlying disease is responsible. If so, it can be addressed separately, and effective treatment to rebuild bone can begin.

Obstructive Sleep Apnea

Breaking News: Sleep is Dangerous!

Is nothing sacred? Obstructive Sleep Apnea (Apnea means "not breathing") is the mechanical restriction of our airway when throat muscles go slack during deep sleep. The result is often loud snoring with periods of no air movement at all into the lungs. First the uvula and soft palate (the soft part of the roof of the mouth) collapse back against the upper airway followed by a limp tongue, which adds its mass. This forms a one-way blockage that allows air to leave but not enter the lungs.

The effort of trying to inhale only causes the blockage to seal more tightly. The brain will not tolerate this nonsense for more than about a minute. It freaks out when blood oxygen drops and carbon dioxide increases, stimulating the ever-increasing urgency for air.

In deep sleep, most muscles relax to the point of paralysis, refreshing themselves for the demands of the coming day. But air is more important than high-quality sleep. The brain quickly abandons the deep sleep state and moves to a much lighter zone. This brings all the muscles back on line to cough, choke, snort, turn over, or do whatever is needed to re-open that airway. Thanks brain!

For the most part, a sleeper remembers none of this, even though it may happen several hundred times every night. They wake with the vague impression of having had a busy, busy night. It's no wonder these people can remain tired after ten hours of sleep and will stumble through the day wondering what on earth is wrong with them.

For most people with obstructive sleep apnea, treatment usually translates into a vastly improved *quality* of life, not necessarily a longer one. It is by no means a high-volume killer, but it is a killer. It earned its place on the Stupid Reasons People Die list, because it is so darn easy to identify and treat.

As many as 25 million Americans have this disorder, yet only about 1 million of them know it. About 15 percent of American males and 4 percent of females are affected. It is likely to strike men in middle age, and hits both elderly men and women. It can also affect children.

The danger is in several areas. One common symptom of sleep apnea is chronic exhaustion with a touch of narcolepsy. Falling asleep at the wheel is much more common in this group, obviously a huge danger for the patient and anyone unlucky enough to be on the road with them.

The next danger is more insidious. With each episode of apnea, the resulting low oxygen levels cause a bit of direct injury to the lung. Over many years, this injury can cause significant destruction to the lung's blood vessels. If you recall, *all* of our blood passes this way every minute or so. Fewer healthy blood vessels means a traffic jam, high blood pressure in the lungs, which causes a destructive strain on the right side of the heart as it struggles to pump against it. Ergo, deadly conditions known as pulmonary hypertension and right-sided heart failure. This means slow suffocation, a particularly bad way to die.

Strokes, heart attacks, abnormal heart rhythms, uncontrollable high blood pressure, and worsening diabetes all contribute to a shorter life expectancy. And all of these occur more commonly in patients with sleep apnea. To name a few of the psychosocial consequences of this condition, there's depression, memory loss, irritability, low sex drive, headaches, and chronic fatigue. Any one of these can make life miserable.

Sometimes, patients are misdiagnosed with ADHD when the real culprit is sleep apnea. It's important to rule out sleep apnea before assigning any psychiatric diagnosis.

Many patients with sleep apnea are overweight, which sets up the mechanical problems that occur during sleep. There are also facial features more commonly found in such patients including thick necks, a narrow upper jaw, a receding chin, overbite, or a larger tongue.

While the "classic" sleep apnea patient might be described as a stocky, no-neck linebacker, it can also occur in 98-pound women with small chins. Men with the disorder are more likely to snore for ten hours every night, while women will often have difficulty getting to sleep each night and suffer mild insomnia.

One reason it's so poorly recognized is the patient sleeps through the whole thing. They may not even recognize how rotten they feel compared to the energy level they once had. If they do, they may blame it on not being as young as "back in the day."

If a sleep apnea patient is lucky, he or she sleeps with someone who knows the difference between a bit of snoring and the fight-for-air variety. Screening starts out very easily, with a short questionnaire like the one below:

Basic Screening for Sleep Apnea:

▶ **Do you snore loudly?**

▶ **Are you overweight?**

▶ **Does your snoring wake you up at night?**

▶ **Do you or your partner notice that you make gasping and choking noises during sleep?**

▶ **Do you have a dry mouth, sore throat or headache in the morning?**

▶ **Do you find it hard to stay awake watching TV, reading a book, or attending a meeting?**

▶ **Are you often irritable, fatigued or have trouble concentrating?**

▶ **Do you have high blood pressure?**

▶ **Do you ever wake up choking, gasping for air, or have a skipping or racing heartbeat?**

If you answered yes to three or more of these questions, you may be suffering from sleep apnea and need further evaluation. If you have any questions about appropriate referrals, check http://www.sleepapnea.org.

Referral to a sleep center is required to evaluate patients. Sleep apnea comes in all shapes, sizes, and levels of severity. In some cases, simple tricks to keep the sleeper off their back, or modest weight loss can make a huge difference. For others, a way to keep the airway open at night must be found.

Continuous positive airway pressure (CPAP) machines and related devices are becoming commonplace as the preferred, non-surgical way to keep the air flowing all night long.

They include a facial mask worn in bed, which is connected to an air source that applies enough pressure to maintain an open airway. One complaint has been that the machines are cumbersome and too much like a hospital respirator. Okay, they aren't exactly sexy, but neither is snoring like a jackhammer. Even less sexy is dying from heart-lung failure. And the improvement in the patient's life can be well worth dealing with the device.

Finally, there are surgical options. I only consider these when the problem is clearly dangerous, and nothing else has worked. If the patient is obese, surgery can be performed to lower weight, such as with a gastric bypass or a gastric banding procedure. However, sleep apnea surgery is usually directed at the neck, jaw, and oral cavity, never a pleasant prospect. Fortunately, the need for surgery is very rare, because most cases can be easily treated.

"Just pretend you're advocating for your child or other loved one instead of yourself, and it's suddenly easier."

Chapter 22
In Closing

So often, we are our own worst enemies. Preconceived ideas of health and disease; natural and chemical; benefit and risk; standard of care and the latest advancements; and who should be responsible for the scope, content, and cost of healthcare translates into shorter lives. Unnecessarily shorter lives.

Our thinking blinds us to making informed, reasoned decisions. Our tendency to choose denial keeps us from taking essential action when we suspect something is wrong. And our habit of accepting news headlines as the truth, the whole truth, and nothing but the truth, leaves us making grave mistakes about maintaining or restoring our health.

Like everything in life, science and technology have dark sides, but remaining uninformed under the assumption that they are all dark is a kind of death wish.

The large gap between an outdated *standard of care* and *state of the art* in health screening, prevention, and treatment, seems to be as wide as ever. Financial, cultural, and healthcare systems seem designed to keep the two as far apart as possible, so that only the most enlightened and determined make it across from one side to the other.

So many people walk around with ticking time bombs, because they refuse to pay for a level of care that would defuse them.

Life is a risk. There are no perfect tools or treatments, no money back guarantees in medicine. Preventive efforts, like screening, can be a double-edged sword. Uncertain results can produce anxiety. An overly-aggressive response to results can be costly and invasive.

Accept the limitations of modern medicine, if you can, and start working on how you can use what we have to benefit you most. We have a lot to work with. And, when necessary, be willing to write a check or pull out the plastic without hesitation, knowing that there are indeed plenty of medical tests and state-of-the-art treatments worth paying for.

Here again, are screening tools that are worth your consideration, time and money. The recommendations below are general guidelines only and should always be discussed with your doctor.

Ultra Fast CT Scan of the Heart

Also called Electron Beam CT Scan (EBCT) or rapid multi-detector CT, these machines see hardening of the arteries. The score on this exam correlates very closely with the risk of heart attack in the next ten years. Ultra Fast CT opens a critical door to preventing a leading cause of early death.

Recommendations: Men over 40 and women over 50. Sooner, if there are other significant risk factors.

Extended Lipid Testing

Lipoprotein particles, the "floating containers" for cholesterol and triglycerides, come in all different shapes and sizes. The state of the art in treating patients with either known heart disease or an EBCT result revealing hardening of the arteries, relies on understanding not only a patient's cholesterol, good and bad, but also the size, shape, and oxidation state of these particles. It is used to individualize treatment plans that reduce risk for heart attack and stroke.

Recommendations: For any person with signs or symptoms of coronary heart disease or cerebrovascular disease. These include heart attack, stroke, angina, TIA (transient ischemic attack) or "near-stroke," coronary artery bypass surgery, coronary angioplasty, or stent placement. Also, recommendations for those with evidence of coronary plaque on Ultra Fast CT Scan or imaging studies that reveal atherosclerosis. Review these laboratory results with a heart specialist.

Ultrasound of the Abdomen

This benign and inexpensive study is highly sensitive in detecting aortic aneurysms, which are now being recognized as a major cause of preventable death. The test has the occasional benefit of finding other problems such as kidney cancers when they are small and detectable, as well as liver and gall bladder disease. It uses no dangerous radiation, costs about $200, and is completely painless.

Recommendations: Complete abdominal ultrasound (not just a quick screen of the aorta) for all men and women, age 40 and over, every four years with appropriate—but usually conservative—followup of any detected abnormalities.

Ultra Fast CT Scan of the Lung

Lung cancer still kills most people who get it, even when found as early as possible by conventional x-rays. Earlier detection is more likely with Ultra Fast CT Scanning. This could turn the tide for high-risk patients—smokers and ex-smokers.

Recommendations: Studies are still underway at this writing, so Ultra Fast CT as a lung cancer screen is entirely optional. The upside: I've known several patients with tumors that were discovered very early. The downside: it involves a moderate dose of radiation, and all cancer screenings must be performed on a regular basis to be effective. How frequently the scan should be done for lung cancer has yet to be decided, but, over time, multiple scans could deliver a fair dose of radiation. It costs a couple hundred dollars.

Colonoscopy

A single colonoscopy can be one of the most life-saving tests you can undergo. Colon cancer is common and sneaky, and no physician can say you will not get it. Yes, it's slow-growing, but it can creep up on you. Colonoscopy can find these tumors when they are small, even *pre*-malignant, and, at the same time, they can be removed. That sure beats major surgery. You may feel there are indignities with the test, but to my knowledge no one has ever died of embarrassment. Preparing your colon with a cleansing prep is a drag, but it's one day of your life that can buy you many more.

Recommendations: Just do it. Every man and woman should undergo colonoscopy no later than age 50—considerably sooner for patients with a family history of colon cancer or *familial polyposis syndrome.* If you're adopted, play it safe and start at age 40. Repeat every ten years for followup unless a problem is found, at which time more frequent followup will be scheduled.

PSA Testing and Rectal Exam

Prostate cancer plays a confusing game. The cancer is common, easy to find, and in many cases won't kill the patient, even if left alone.

Every treatment has its pros and cons, including surgery, radiation, cryotherapy, and watchful waiting. Even diagnostic biopsies can be damaging. It's important to be able to deal with uncertainty when choosing to be screened for this cancer. However, I believe screening is the wise thing to do. Handling abnormal results is a complex subject. Take another look at Chapter 19, and check our website for updates and new developments.

Recommendations: Guys, have your PSA level checked every year after age 40, and add annual rectal exams starting at age 50.

Mammogram and MRI of the Breast

Breast cancer is the scourge of modern women. Although there's a great deal of public awareness, many women, especially of low socioeconomic status, fail to be screened, and many women are not aware of the rare and deadly form known as Inflammatory Breast Cancer (IBC). Breast cancer runs in families, and several genetic markers have been discovered. This allows identification of a subset of women who are at especially high risk. For this group, in addition to mammography, additional testing with the more sensitive MRI scanner may be indicated. This is especially true for young women with denser breast tissue or who have implants. In these cases, mammography is not as effective at detecting abnormalities.

Recommendations: Know your breasts. Weekly self-examination starting at age 18. Note any changes of any kind. Initial mammogram at age 35, another at age 38, and every year after age 40 for all women.

MRI scanning as well for women at high risk as defined by a strong family history and/or based on results of genetic testing as early as 30 years of age. Immediate mammogram and other testing, as needed, for a suspicious new lump, pucker, or leak. Know about Inflammatory Breast Cancer (IBC), and act immediately when you find signs, symptoms, or anything that raises your concern.

Regular Skin Checks

The beauty mark from hell, Malignant Melanoma, is usually in plain sight. But some people have hundreds of dark moles, creating a perfect camouflage. It may require a trained eye to find a problem. Regular inspection of your skin is all the high-tech screening needed to catch the majority of these cancers.

Recommendations: Make skin awareness a way of life. Do a quick check when bathing. If you're fortunate enough to share your life with another, watch each other's back. Keep an eye on your partner's hard-to-see places including their scalp, neck, back and rear. See your physician or a dermatologist at least once a year for a complete body skin check, and if you have Dysplastic Nevus Syndrome (hundreds of flat, dark moles), talk to a dermatologist about a photo survey of your skin.

Pill Cameras and Endoscopes

When stomach acid goes where is shouldn't, bad things happen. It should not visit your esophagus. With the obesity epidemic in our nation, gastric reflux is becoming more and more common. Throw alcohol and tobacco abuse into the mix, and it's understandable that esophageal cancer is one of the fastest growing cancers in our country.

People with symptoms of reflux or just chronic heartburn should have an endoscopy to directly inspect and sample tissue in the lower esophagus.

About 40 percent of the time, the reflux is there but the heartburn isn't. For those who want a quick look without losing a day to sedation, the PillCam® offers a fast, painless, and virtually risk-free view.

Recommendations: I recommend this procedure *electively* as a screen for people over 50 who have had *no significant symptoms* of heartburn or reflux, especially if they have been a smoker, heavy drinker, or are obese. How frequently it should be done has not yet been determined. I currently consider once every ten years up to age 80 as a reasonable, if somewhat arbitrary, schedule. It's definitely *not* for the patient who's already symptomatic with heartburn. They need the gold standard of endoscopy. PillCam® costs a lot, $1200 to $1500, and most patients will be writing that check themselves.

Urine Cytology

Bladder cancer can be found earlier by employing a skilled profes-sional to look for abnormal cells in the urine. Abnormal cells can be missed, even when present, but when combined with the common Urine Analysis test for blood, it offers a better early warning system. We don't yet know if this means a higher survival rate for bladder cancer, but the only down-side is the cost, currently about $45 per year.

Recommendations: Once a year, no later than age 40, add Urine Cytology to the Urine Analysis test that most patients receive as part of the annual physical.

Ovarian Cancer Screening

We're just not there yet. For this rare cancer with lots of mostly false-positive screening results, widespread screening is likely to do more harm than good at this time. But stay tuned, breakthroughs are overdue, and some promising results are hitting the medical literature at this writing. For women at high risk, those with one or more first-degree relatives with the disease, screening probably makes sense.

Recommendations: Annual CA-125 blood test for *high-risk* women with transvaginal ultrasound as part of the annual gynecological exam. Be prepared for the potential of a false-positive test result. If this kind of accelerated screening is too stressful for an individual, she's probably better off without it.

PAP Smear and HPV Vaccination

Doctors live for the kind of progress we've made against cervical cancer, an 80 percent decrease in deaths since PAP Smear screening was introduced. Gynecological testing remains vital to discover this cancer years before it can hurt us. The use of the new vaccine against Human Papilloma Virus, Gardasil, will help launch a new generation of women protected against the cause of almost all cervical cancer.

Recommendations: Schedule annual PAP smears, and show up for them. Girls and women between the ages of nine and twenty-six are candidates for a three-dose course of a vaccine that may save their lives. The information about this vaccine is still too new to know if older women would benefit from vaccination or if boosters will be needed after many years. It's new. There could always be some future media frenzy about undiscovered side-effects, but they would have to be pretty deadly to outweigh the benefits of slashing the cervical cancer rate. I believe the argument that such a vaccine encourages destructive sexual behavior and removes an appropriate "natural consequence" of such behavior is idiotic.

DEXA Scan Screening for Osteoporosis

Thin bones kill. *All* women are susceptible to osteopenia (thin bones) and osteoporosis (very thin bones) after menopause. Since Mother Nature didn't plan on us living once we can no longer reproduce, 90 percent of a woman's estrogen disappears forever after age 50. This leads to bone mineral loss.

Men lose bone mass as well, though usually later in life. DEXA Scan screening is easy, and treatments today are highly effective in restoring bone mineral and reducing deadly fractures.

Recommendations: DEXA scan for all women at age 50 and all men starting at age 60, (although "official" recommendations for men will likely be set at a later age.) Followup exams should be scheduled as needed based on the results. Those with conditions known to place them at higher risk should screen earlier.

Breathe When You're Sleeping

A mechanical disorder that interferes with breathing during sleep can be detected, in many cases, with a simple questionnaire. Obstructive Sleep Apnea screening requires spending a night in a sleep lab where the details of each patient's disorder and treatment can be worked out. Failure to find and treat this common problem can lead to a diminished quality of life from chronic deprivation of *deep* sleep. It can kill from chronic hypoxic (low oxygen) injury to the lungs and heart, not to mention the risk of a fatal automobile accident due to severe daytime drowsiness.

Recommendations: Fill out a Sleep Apnea Questionnaire. Ask your partner or a family member about your snoring and if you hold your breath during sleep. Seek help at a qualified sleep clinic if you have symptoms!

After the Screening?

If a cancer is found, the response is usually easy: get rid of it. Our biggest killer, atherosclerosis, requires a more subtle approach. Cutting out damaged arteries to our hearts and brains is not an option. We must identify *all* the factors likely to be contributing to each patient's problem, considering everything from Metabolic Syndrome, the size and shape of our cholesterol particles, diabetes, hypertension, and many others, and then treat each one effectively.

This requires the help of specialists, the best medications available, and knowledge of the state-of-the-art treatment for preventing heart attacks and strokes. Frankly, it also requires an aggressive attitude on the part of the physician. Coronary artery disease is not an area for "wait and watch" medicine.

Sleep apnea, thin bones? Treat them.

I urge you to be a dedicated player in your own healthcare. In fact, you should be the team leader. No one is more qualified to call the shots about you than you. It's not hard. Concise and accurate information is available to help you work with your healthcare providers to decide your best strategies for living longer.

You might need to get pushy once in a while. Just pretend you're advocating for your child or other loved one instead of yourself, and it's suddenly easier. Be willing to back up the plan by staying current on health issues that are relevant to you, and be willing to invest some of your earnings to get the best possible care.

Hey, it's your life.

You're smart enough to look after it.

APPENDICES

Appendix 1

U.S. Preventive Services Task Force (USPSTF)

This description of the USPSTF is directly from the *Agency for Healthcare Research and Quality* web page: http://www.ahrq.gov/clinic/uspstfix.htm#About

The U.S. Preventive Services Task Force is an independent panel of experts in primary care and prevention that systematically reviews the evidence of effectiveness and develops recommendations for clinical preventive services. Sponsored since 1998 by the Agency for Healthcare Research and Quality (AHRQ), the Task Force is the leading independent panel of private-sector experts in prevention and primary care. For each condition being considered, a USPSTF committee will review the available information, assess the quality of that information (good, fair, poor), and assign one of five ratings or recommendations, reflecting the strength of evidence and magnitude of net benefit (benefits minus harms):

Strength of Recommendations

Rating **A:** The USPSTF strongly recommends that clinicians provide the service to eligible patients. The USPSTF found good evidence that the service improves important health outcomes and concludes that benefits substantially outweigh harms.

Rating **B:** The USPSTF recommends that clinicians provide this service to eligible patients. The USPSTF found at least fair evidence that the service improves important health outcomes and concludes that benefits outweigh harms.

Rating **C:** The USPSTF makes no recommendation for or against routine provision of the service. The USPSTF found at least fair evidence that the service can improve health outcomes but concludes that the balance of benefits and harms is too close to justify a general recommendation.

Rating **D:** The USPSTF recommends against routinely providing the service to asymptomatic patients. The USPSTF found at least fair evidence that the service is ineffective or that harms outweigh benefits.

Rating **I:** The USPSTF concludes that the evidence is insufficient to recommend for or against routinely providing the service. Evidence that the service is effective is lacking, of poor quality, or conflicting, and the balance of benefits and harms cannot be determined.

Strength of Evidence

Good: Evidence includes consistent results from well-designed, well-conducted studies in representative populations that directly assess effects on health outcomes.

Fair: Evidence is sufficient to determine effects on health outcomes, but the strength of the evidence is limited by the number, quality, or consistency of the individual studies, generalizability to routine practice, or indirect nature of the evidence on health outcomes.

Poor: Evidence is insufficient to assess the effects on health outcomes because of limited number or power of studies, important flaws in their design or conduct, gaps in the chain of evidence, or lack of information on important health outcomes.

Appendix 2

Atherosclerotic Plaque Morphology

Atherosclerotic plaques do indeed contain lots of cholesterol, but they also contain much more. It turns out that cholesterol is a vital part of our bodies and, like oxygen and glucose, must be transported around the body in our bloodstream. However, since it is essentially like oil, it cannot dissolve in water. It therefore travels inside microscopic "vehicles," complexes of fats, proteins, and polysaccharides that can dissolve in the blood and thereby be easily transported. One such vehicle, the Low Density Lipoprotein Complex (or LDL cholesterol as it's commonly called), is designed to distribute cholesterol and other forms of lipids (oily or fatty molecules) to the various tissues that need them. They are small enough to penetrate throughout many tissues, and that includes the artery walls.

However, once there, they sometimes meet up with a patrolling white blood cell called a macrophage, the soldiers of the immune system, which decides to eat the cholesterol, especially if it has undergone a process called oxidation. If it eats enough, it decides to stay put and stop patrolling, getting fatter and fatter. It is now called a "foam cell," and it's not ever planning to leave.

When enough of these cells do this, we have the beginning of a plaque. As it grows, the plaque forms a complex structure of these foam cells plus fibrous tissue and some muscle cells, presumably borrowed from the normal muscle cells surrounding the artery. This becomes a full-grown plaque complete with many transformed macrophage foam cells, a cholesterol "core" and a "cap." The cap is that part just under the endothelium, the inner lining of the artery, and it seems to make all the difference when it comes to the likelihood of a plaque rupture. If the cap is strongly built, with muscle cells that add stability, the plaque is likely to be "stable."

However, if the cap is lacking such structural strength, instead being constructed of looser fibrous tissue, it may not provide adequate strength to stand up against the constant stress of high-pressure blood flow. It's a bit of a real-life straw house versus brick house situation. A major difference between stable and unstable plaques has to do with the activity of the white blood cells they contain. Among the many biologic processes that occur, these cells secrete enzymes known as metalloproteases, which can tear apart other molecules. They tend to be more active near the edges of the plaques (the "shoulder" region) where the cap is thinnest and there is little structural support.

This inflammation, the presence of metabolically-active white blood cells and all the chemistry they set in motion, thereby undermines the integrity of the plaque structure and increases the chance of rupture. This would then expose the passing blood and its platelets to the underlying plaque and its lipids, and an obstructing blood clot, a thrombus, could form causing a heart attack. This is the reason that halting inflammation in a plaque is considered to be a key element in the strategy to prevent heart attacks.

Appendix 3

Framingham Cardiac Risk Assessment Tools

The likelihood that you will suffer a heart attack can be very accurately predicted. This type of information, however, is more useful to predict the outcome for groups of people than for individuals. The nature of the statistic is to predict what percentage of a group, with certain measured risk traits, will still be alive and well after a given period of time, and how many won't. The trouble for an individual is that we have no way of knowing which members of the group will survive and which will fall. Nonetheless, it has been useful to rank individuals according to the risk assigned to their respective groups in order to help us decide who should undergo aggressive therapy to lower their risk, and who can be spared the most aggressive treatments.

The scoring relies on these traits for each individual:

▶ **age**
▶ **gender**
▶ **blood pressure**
▶ **LDL Cholesterol level**
▶ **HDL Cholesterol level**
▶ **Presence or absence of Diabetes**
▶ **Presence or absence of smoking**

A usable worksheet was impractical to print in this book but they can be easily found and downloaded from the internet. One location providing them at the time of this writing is the website of The National Heart Lung and Blood Institute http://www.nhlbi.nih.gov/about/framingham/riskabs.htm. An online interactive Framingham Assessment calculator is also available through the Medical College of Wisconsin web page: http://www.intmed.mcw.edu/clincalc/heartrisk.html

Appendix 4

BMI: Body Mass Index of Obesity

Obesity: definitions and BMI calculators

The level of normal weight, up to overweight, and on into obesity is typically measured on a scale from about 16 to 45. This definition from the Centers for Disease Control and Prevention (CDC) describes the system used most widely in the United States:

> *Overweight and obesity are both labels for ranges of weight that are greater than what is generally considered healthy for a given height. The terms also identify ranges of weight that have been shown to increase the likelihood of certain diseases and other health problems. For adults, overweight and obesity ranges are determined by using weight and height to calculate a number called the "body mass index" (BMI). BMI is used because, for most people, it correlates with their amount of body fat. An adult who has a BMI between 25 and 29.9 is considered over-weight. An adult who has a BMI of 30 or higher is considered obese.*

Several websites offer an automatic calculator to help you deter-mine your body mass index, and some offer software downloads to do the same from your own handheld computer. This page at National Heart Lung and Blood Institute (NHLBI) will give you a quick result: http://www.nhlbisupport.com/bmi/.

This CDC page offers one for adults *and* children: http://www.cdc.gov/nccdphp/dnpa/bmi/index.htm.

This page, also at the NHLBI site, offers a download to use on a handheld computer, very handy for healthcare providers of all kinds: http://hp2010.nhlbihin.net/bmi_palm.htm.

It's also easy to calculate BMI by hand if the internet isn't handy. Here's how:

Calculating the BMI is simple. We just take our weight and divide it by the square of our height, which is WEIGHT / (HEIGHT x HEIGHT) = Body Mass Index. The math formula looks like this $BMI=Wt(kg)/(Ht(M))^2$

The inconvenient part for us non-metric folks is that first we must know the values for our weight in *Kilograms* instead of in pounds and the values for our height in *meters* instead of in feet and inches. Here's how:

First, write down your weight in pounds and multiply it by 0.45. The result is your weight in kilograms. Write the result down, label it as "my weight" and set it aside.

Next, write down your height in feet, leaving out the inches for now (for example, if you are 5 feet 3-½ inches, just write down the '5'). Multiply this number by 0.305. Write down this result, label it as "height part 1" and set it aside.

Next, write down your extra height inches (in our example of the 5 foot 3-½ inch person, you would just write down the '3.5'). Multiply this by the number 0.0254, and label the result "height part 2." Next add "height part 1" and "height part 2" together and label the result "my height."

Finally, to calculate your BMI simply divide "my weight" by the square of "my height" (the square of "my height" is: "my height" x "my height") to get your BMI.

BMI = "my weight" / ("my height" x "my height")

For example: Mary is 5 foot 3-½ inches and weighs 141 pounds. We will round off values containing more than three significant digits.

Mary's **weight** is 141 x 0.45 = 63.45 we'll round off to: **63.5** (kilograms)
Mary's **height part 1** is 5 x 0.305 = 1.525 we'll round off to **1.53** (meters) and Mary's **height part 2** is 3.5 x 0.0254 = 0.0889 we'll round off to **0.089** (meters).
Mary's **total height** is 1.53 + .089 = **1.619** (meters).

Mary's BMI is calculated by dividing her weight by the square of her height. So let's calculate the square of her height: total height squared is 1.619 x 1.619 = 2.621 (rounded to **2.62**) meters squared. Finally, her weight divided by the square of her height becomes 63.5/2.62 = 24.23 kilograms per meter squared or **24.23 kg/m2.** Mary's BMI is pretty normal!

Appendix 5

Lipoprotein [a]

Lipoprotein [a]—abbreviated Lp[a], is essentially a modified LDL particle (see Appendix 2) circulating in the bloodstream. The structure of the Lp[a] particle is very similar to a normal LDL particle linked to a plasminogen molecule. (Plasminogen is involved in dissolving blood clots.) The function of Lp[a] is unknown.

It is *associated* with the development of atherosclerosis; people with high levels of Lp[a] are definitely at an elevated risk of this kind of heart disease. But whether Lp[a] is directly involved in the atherosclerotic process or is just a barometer of *something else* that is toxic has yet to be determined.

Treatments to lower Lp[a] are limited. Nicotinic acid (Niacin) has been shown to lower concentration of Lp[a] to some small degree as does estrogen supplementation, but we do not know if direct treatment to lower it is helpful in preventing heart attacks or strokes.

Current use of Lp[a] as a test marker revolves around determining the *intensity* of therapy for LDL cholesterol in general. In the presence of elevated Lp[a], there is evidence that LDL cholesterol should be treated more aggressively, so we might lower the targets for our LDL cholesterol levels.

Appendix 6

Breast Cancer Risk and Screening Guidelines

The formula to estimate risk for breast cancer is complex and is best performed by computer. An interactive breast cancer risk assessment tool can be found at this page of the National Cancer Institute website http://www.cancer.gov/bcrisktool/ and at this website by Steven B. Halls, MD, http://www.halls.md/breast/risk.htm.

Screening Recommendations:

Cancer screening recommendations differ between various organizations. Included here are those of The American Cancer Society (ACS), which are the same as those of the Susan G. Komen Breast Cancer Foundation for the general population. They are followed by those of the ACS for high-risk women:

> *"Breast Self-Exam beginning in 20s, review benefits and limitations of self-exam with health care provider. Choice to perform self-exam is up to individual. Clinical Breast Exam by well-woman provider at least every 3 years between ages 20-39. Mammography is recommended every year beginning at age 40."*

Women at high risk have more aggressive recommendations:

> *"A person who carries either the BRCA1 or BRCA2 mutation OR who have two or more first-degree relatives with a history of breast OR Ovarian cancer should perform monthly self-exam and obtain a clinical breast exam every year from age 20 to 25, then twice a year thereafter. Annual mammograms should also start at age 25 in this group."*

Other resources include the Susan G. Komen Breast Cancer Foundation at http://www.komen.org for general breast cancer information and the Inflammatory Breast Cancer Research Foundation at http://www.ibcresearch.org/.

Appendix 7

MRI vs. Mammogram in High Risk Patients

Statistics From Chapter 20: *Is Mammogram the best we've got?*

In this Dutch study on high-risk women, invasive breast cancer was correctly diagnosed more often with MRI. These statistics can be a bit confusing, but I want to list them here for those who like to know the numbers:

	Sensitivity	Specificity
Breast Exam:	17.9%	98.1%
Mammogram:	33.3%	95.0%
MRI:	79.5%	89.8%

▶ **There were a total of 1909 women followed; all had both MRI and Mammogram annually.**

▶ **MRI picked up 32 cancers but missed 13 of them.**

▶ **Mammogram picked up 18 cancers but missed 27 of them.**

▶ **Of the 32 cancers picked up by MRI, Mammogram missed 22 of them.**

▶ **Of the 22 cancers picked up by Mammogram, MRI missed 13 of them.**

▶ **Of the 13 cancers missed by MRI, 8 were picked up by Mammogram.**

▶ **Of the 27 cancers missed by Mammogram, 22 were picked up by MRI.**

Appendix 8

Positron Emission Tomography (PET) Scan Information

Positron Emission Tomography Scanning is an imaging technique capable of detecting small areas of increased metabolic activity, as in cancer, or of outlining areas of dramatically reduced metabolic activity, such as in the brain stricken with Alzheimer Disease.

Since metabolic activity means consumption of both oxygen and a fuel source such as glucose, we can introduce radioactive oxygen or glucose, into the body (a tracer) where it can be expected to concentrate faster in areas of higher metabolism. The use of oxygen as a tracer is often impractical due to the short half-life of its radioactive isotope. However, analogs of glucose and other fuels can be prepared with the more useful radioactive properties needed.

The most common radio-tracer in use today is 18F-fluorodeoxyglucose (18F-FDG), a sugar molecule that is recognized as glucose by many body tissues. When this unstable molecule decays, it emits a positron, essentially an antimatter electron, which interacts almost immediately with a regular electron, both of which are thereby annihilated. In this high-energy reaction, two high-energy photons are released, which speed away from each other at 180 degrees, making it possible for a detector to localize their origin along the straight line of their path. Measure tens of thousands of these photons coming in all directions from a tumor or other source of high tracer concentration, and the Pet Scanner can form a computerized image of where in the body the activity originates.

PET is used heavily in medical oncology for medical imaging of tumors and the search for metastases, and in human brain and heart research. It has the ability to do more than take a "snapshot" of the body; it can be used to measure the change in metabolism or blood flow in tissues over time, making it particularly useful in the study of dynamic processes such as the "evolution" of a migraine headache, or the difference in "thinking" between average individuals and those with ADHD, or with actual mental illness.

Of course, there are limitations.

The isotope is short-lived and, until recently, scanners had to be located near the cyclotron that creates the tracer. Most scanners are whole body scanners, making them not only big and expensive, but less accurate for resolving images of small lesions. The more tissue through which a high-energy photon must pass, the more likely it is that one or the other of a pair will be stopped before it reaches the detector ring outside the patient. This leads to inaccuracies that can limit image resolution.

The availability of radio-tracer via distribution centers has improved, and the construction of smaller scanners designed for specific body areas makes this a promising technology for breast and other cancer screenings in the future.

Appendix 9

The ABCDE Criteria in Malignant Melanoma

The "ABCDE" method has proven useful in evaluating skin lesions as possible malignant melanoma. The mnemonic is easily remembered by physicians and laypersons alike. The letters stand for:

Asymmetry: One-half of the lesion does not match the other half.

Border irregularity: The edges are ragged, notched, or blurred.

Color variation: The pigmentation is not uniform and may display shades of tan, brown, or black; white, reddish, or blue discoloration is of particular concern.

Diameter: A diameter greater than 6 mm is characteristic, although some melanomas may have smaller diameters; any growth in a nevus warrants an evaluation.

Evolving: Changes in the lesion over time are characteristic; this factor is critical for nodular or amelanotic (non-pigmented) melanoma, which may not exhibit the classic criteria above.

The ABCDEs have the greatest accuracy when used in combination. Lesions exhibiting all these features should be considered potential melanoma, and the absence of one or two feature should *not* stop anyone from seeking a professional evaluation. In fact, a forth letter, F, has been suggested in the literature for *any* Funny-Looking mole.

Appendix 10

Cervical Cancer Screening Guidelines

These are the Cervical Cancer Screening Guidelines currently recommended by the America Cancer Society as of this writing:

> *All women should begin cervical cancer screening about 3 years after they begin having vaginal intercourse, but no later than when they are 21 years old. Screening should be done every year with the regular Pap test or every 2 years using the newer liquid-based Pap test.*
>
> *Beginning at age 30, women who have had 3 normal Pap test results in a row may get screened every 2 to 3 years. Another reasonable option for women over 30 is to get screened every 3 years (but not more frequently) with either the conventional or liquid-based Pap test, plus the HPV DNA test. Women who have certain risk factors, such as diethylstilbestrol (DES) exposure before birth, HIV infection, or a weakened immune system due to organ transplant, chemotherapy, or chronic steroid use, should continue to be screened annually.*
>
> *Women 70 years of age or older who have had 3 or more normal Pap tests in a row and no abnormal Pap test results in the last 10 years may choose to stop having cervical cancer screening. Women with a history of cervical cancer, DES exposure before birth, HIV infection or a weakened immune system, should continue to have screening as long as they are in good health.*
>
> *Women who have had a total hysterectomy (removal of the uterus and cervix) may also choose to stop having cervical cancer screening, unless the surgery was done as a treatment for cervical cancer or precancer. Women who have had a hysterectomy without removal of the cervix should continue to follow the guidelines above.*

Appendix 11

Gleason Scoring

Let's begin with what the Gleason Score is and what it *isn't*. This is a method to *grade*, not to *stage* prostate cancer. Staging is determining how far a tumor has spread; in other words, is it contained within the original organ, or has it already set up shop throughout the body?

Grading is a measurement of how aggressive the tumor cells *appear* in the microscope. In general, the closer to normal tissue malignant cells appear, the less aggressively they behave. In the case of prostate cancer, a pathologist reviews either small tissue samples after biopsy or the entire prostate gland after its surgical removal.

The Gleason score was developed in 1966 by pathologist Dr. Donald Gleason. Although it's yet another statistical estimate of how a population will behave being forced upon the individual cancer patient, it has been remarkably useful to urologists for four decades. The grading system has two unique features. First, it considers only the architectural pattern, not the cellular features of the tumor. Second, the pathologist does not look for the worst of all the cancer cell types he or she sees but rather the most common pattern they see.

This just isn't how things are generally done in cancer grading, but as we saw in Chapter 19, prostate cancer behaves sometimes as a low-grade annoyance and sometimes as an aggressive invader. Dr. Gleason realized each tumor could have multiple personalities and demonstrated that the best predictor of the tumor's future behavior came from discovering which architectural patterns dominated within the tumor.

These architectural features (see diagram) are separated into five general patterns, 1 being the most like normal tissue and, therefore, at lowest level of aggression, and 5 being the most bizarre. The most prevalent *and* the second most prevalent pattern are identified, and the number score of each is added together. For example, if 40% of the tumor appears to be pattern 2, and 30% is pattern 4, the score becomes $2 + 4 = 6$.

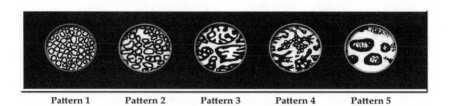

Pattern 1   Pattern 2   Pattern 3   Pattern 4   Pattern 5

Total scores range, obviously, from 2 to 10 and are broken down into three general levels:

▶ **Low-grade (well-differentiated) tumors, have a score of 4 or less.**

▶ **Intermediate-grade (moderately differentiated), somewhere between the low- and high-grade cancers, is the most common range with a score of between 4 and 7. These tumors can behave overall like either a high- or low-grade cancer. Much depends on other factors such as PSA level and tumor volume.**

▶ **High-grade (poorly-differentiated) tumors, have scores from 8 to 10. These are the most deadly, often aggressive, and fast-growing.**

Of course, it's possible to get the same score in several different ways. If a patient's total score is 4 + 3 = 7, this means the *predominant* pattern was a 4 and the next in line was pattern 3. A different patient could also get a score of 7, but like this: 3 + 4 = 7, wherein the most prevalent pattern is the less aggressive pattern 3. If a pretty large fraction of pattern 5 cells are found to take the third position, this should also be noted when interpreting the score and using it to gauge the appropriate level of therapy.

Bibliography

General

Dawkins, Richard. **The Selfish Gene,** Oxford University Press, 1989

Eker, T Harv. **Secrets of the Millionaire Mind** *Mastering the Game of Inner Wealth,* Collins (February 15, 2005)

Gladwell, Malcolm. **Blink:** *The Power of Thinking Without Thinking,* Malcolm Gladwell Little, Brown and Company (January 11, 2005)

[1] Harris, Sam. **The End of Faith:** *Religion, Terror and the Future of Reason,* Norton, W.W. Norton & Company, *Inc* in US, *Ltd.* in London. (2005)

Lange, Paul H and Adamec, Christine. *Prostate Cancer For Dummies,* For Dummies; 1st edition (April 1, 2003)

Levitt, Steven D and Dubner, Stephen J. **Freakonomics:** *A Rogue Economist Explores the Hidden Side of Everything,* William Morrow & Co (2005)

[2] Rushkoff, Douglas. **Coercion:** *Why We Listen to What "They" Say,* Riverhead Books, a member of Penguin Putman, Inc. (1999)

Chapter 2

Journal of the American Medical Association. May 21, 2003; Vol 289(19). *The Seventh Report of the Joint National Committee on Prevention, Detection, Evaluation, and Treatment of High Blood Pressure The JNC 7 Report* Aram V Chobanian, MD; George L BakOs, MD; Henry R Black, MD; William C Cushman, MD; Lee A Green, MD, MPH; Joseph L Izzo, Jr, MD; Daniel W Jones, MD; Barry J Materson, MD, MBA; Suzanne Oparil, MD; Jackson T Wright, Jr, MD, PhD; Edward J Roccella, PhD, MPH; and the National High Blood Pressure Education Program Coordinating Committee

National Institute on Alcohol Abuse and Alcoholism website. http://www.niaaa.nih.gov/

Chapter 3

American Journal of Medicine. 2005;118:1087-93. *Lack of Herbal Supplement Characterization in Published Randomized Controlled Trials.* Peter M Wolsko, MD; David K Solondz, BSE; Russell S Phillips, MD; Steven C Schachter, MD; David M Eisenberg, MD

Chapter 5

American Journal of Health-System Pharmacy. 2003;60:1580-82. *Time to ban ephedra—now.* Guharoy and Noviasky

BioMed Central | BMC Cardiovascular Disorders. Jun 11,2003;3:5. (ISSN 1471-2261) *Risk of Valvular Heart Disease Associated With Use of Fenfluramine.* Hopkins PN, Polukoff GI

Chest. Nov 11,2000;118(5):1516-17. *Mortality from primary pulmonary hypertension in the United States, 1979-1996.* Lilienfeld DE, Rubin LJ.

Circulation. Dec 12,2000;102(24):E180. *Prevalence and determinants of valvulopathy in patients treated with dexfenfluramine.* Shively BK, Roldan CA, Gill EA, Najarian T, Loar SB.

Chapter 7

Absolute vs. Relative Risk. from The Foundation For Informed Decision Making

American Journal of Preventive Medicine. 2003;25(2):101-6 (ISSN: 0749-3797). *Autism and thimerosal-containing vaccines: lack of consistent evidence for an association.* Stehr-Green P, Tull P, Stellfeld M, Mortenson PB, Simpson D

Expert Review of Vaccines. 2004;3(1):19-22 (ISSN: 1476-0584). *MMR vaccine and autism: an update of the scientific evidence.* DeStefano F, Thompson WW

Lipidletter. Sept 2005;Vol 5(1). *Statin Safety: Weighing the Evidence.* Antonio M Gotto, Jr. MD; D Phil; Peter Libby, MD

Pediatrics. 2003;112(3)Pt 1:604-6 (ISSN: 1098-4275). *Thimerosal and the occurrence of autism: negative ecological evidence from Danish population-based data.* Madsen KM, Lauritsen MB, Pedersen CB, Thorsen P, Plesner AM, Andersen PH, Mortensen PB

Chapter 8

American College of Physicians. 2006. Annual Session. *Reforming Primary Care: A Comprehensive Strategy From the American College of Physicians.* Richard Glickman-Simon, MD

American Journal of Medicine. 2005;118:1061-63. *Confronting the Brutal Facts in Health Care.* Editorial

Chapter 9

The Atlantic Monthly. April 2006. *The Drug Pushers - As America turns its health-care system over to the market, pharmaceutical reps are wielding more and more influence—and the line between them and the doctor is beginning to blur.* Carl Elliott

Chapter 10

Cleveland Clinic Journal of Medicine. Jan 2004;Vol 71(1):47-56. *Whole-Body CT Screening for Cancer and Coronary Disease; Does It Pass the Test.* Michael T Modic, MD; Nancy Obuchowski, PhD

Chapter 12

A conventional but informative review of the subject of atherosclerosis, its known causes, and its effects. http://health.howstuffworks.com/heart-attack.htm

Home Page to the original Electron Beam technology. http://www.heartscan.com/

Chapter 13

American Journal of Cardiology. Aug 15,2000;Vol 86(4). *Effects of Simvastatin (40 and 80 mg/day) in Patients With Mixed Hyperlipidemia.* Evan Stein, MD, PhD; Diane Plotkin, PhD; Harold Bays, MD; Michael Davidson, MD; Carlos Dujovne, MD; Stanley Korenman, MD; Michael Stepanavage, BS; and Michele Mercuri, MD, PhD

Annals of Internal Medicine. 1993;119:969-976. *Coronary Angiographic Changes with Lovastatin Therapy - The Monitored Atherosclerosis Regression Study (MARS).* David H Blankenhorn MD, Stanley P Azen PhD, Dieter M Kramsch MD, Wendy J Mack PhD, Linda Cashin-Hemphil MD, Howard N Hodis MD, Laurence WV DeBoer MD, Peter R Mahrer MD, Mary Jo Masteller RN, Laura I Vailas MS RD, Petar Alaupovic PhD, Laurence J Hirsch MD and the MARS Research Group

British Journal of Cardiology. Dec 1999;Vol 6(12). *The Impact of Micronized Fenofibrate on Lipid Subfractions and on reaching HDL-target levels in 7,098 patients with dyslipidaemia.* Neil Poulter

Circulation. March 1994;Vol 89(3). *Effects of Monotherapy With an HMG-CoA Reductase Inhibitor On Progression of Coronary Atherosclerosis as Assessed by Serial Quantitative Arteriography - The Canadian Coronary Atherosclerosis Intervention Trial.* David Waters, MD; Lyall Higginson, MD; Peter Gladstone, MD; Brian Kimball, MD; Michel Le May, MD; Stephen J Boccuzzi, PhD; Jacques Lesperance, MD; the CCAIT Study Group

Journal of the American Medical Association. March 3,2004;Vol 291(9): 1071. *Effect of Intensive Compared With Moderate Lipid-Lowering Therapy on Progression of Coronary Atherosclerosis A Randomized Controlled Trial.* Steven E Nissen, MD; E Murat Tuzcu, MD; Paul Schoenhagen, MD; B Greg Brown, MD; Peter Ganz, MD; Robert A Vogel, MD; Tim Crowe, BS; Gail Howard, MS; Christopher J Cooper, MD; Bruce Brodie, MD; Cindy L Grines, MD; Anthony N DeMaria, MD for the REVERSAL Investigators

Lancet. March 23, 2002;Vol 359(9311):1004-10. *Cardiovascular Morbidity and Mortality in Patients With Diabetes in the Losartan Intervention For Endpoint Reduction in Hypertension Study (LIFE): A Randomised Trial Against Atenolol.* Lars H Lindholm, Hans Ibsen, Bjorn Dahlof, Richard B Devereux, Gareth Beevers, Vlf de Faire, Frej Fyhrquist, Stevo Julius, Sverre E Kjeldsen, Krister Kristiansson, Ole Lederballe-Pedersen, Markku S Nieminen, Per Omvik, Suzanne Oparil, Hans Wedel, Peter Aurup, Jonathan Edelman, Steven Snapinn, for the LIFE study group

Lancet. July 6, 2002;Vol 360(9236):7-22. *MRC/BHF Heart Protection Study of Cholesterol Lowering with Simvastatin in 20,536 High-Risk Individuals: A Randomised Placebo-Controlled Trial.* Heart Protection Study Collaborative Group

Lancet. April 5, 2003;Vol 361(9364):1149-58. *Prevention of coronary and stroke events with atorvastatin in hypertensive patients who have average or lower-than-average cholesterol concentrations, in the Anglo-Scandinavian Cardiac Outcomes Trial-Lipid Lowering Arm (ASCOT-LLA): a multicentre randomised controlled trial.* Peter s. Sever, Bjom-Dahlof, Neil R. Poulter, Hans Wedel, Gareth Beevers, Mark Caulkield, Rory Collins, Sverre E. Kjeldsen, Ami Kristifsson, Gordon r Mcinnes, Jesper Mehlsen, Markku Nieminen, Eain O'Brien, Jan Ostergren, for the ASCOT investigators

Lancet. June 14, 2003;Vol 361(9374):2005-16. *MRC/BHF Heart Protection Study of cholesterol-lowering with simvastatin in 5963 people with diabetes: a randomised placebo-controlled trial.* Heart Protection Study Collaborative Group

Lipid Disorders. 2003;Vol 3(1). *Pleiotropic Effects of Arterial Lipoprotein Trafficking: Understanding the Cellular Saboteurs.* David P HalJar, PhD; Antonio M Gotto, Jr., MD; D Phil

Lipidletter. March 2003;Vol 2(3). *Statin Effects Beyond LDL: Emerging Evidence.* Neil L Coplan, MD; Carl J Vaughn, MD

Chapter 14

American Journal of Roentgenology. 2004;182(5):1327-32 (ISSN: 0361-803X). *Evaluating changes in coronary artery calcium: an analytic method that accounts for interscan variability.* Hokanson JE, MacKenzie T, Kinney G, Snell-Bergeon JK, Dabelea D, Ehrlich J, Eckel RH, Rewers M

Archives of Internal Medicine. Mar 26,2001;Vol 161. *Electron-Beam Computed tomography in the Diagnosis of Coronary Artery Disease - a meta-analysis.* Brahmajee K Nallamothu, MD, MPH; Sanjay Saint, MD, MPH; Lawrence F Bielak, DDS, MPH; Seema S Sonnad, PhD; Patricia A Peyser, PhD; Melvyn Rubenfire, MD; A Mark Fendrick MD

Circulation. 1995;92:632-36. *Coronary Artery Screening by Electron Beam Computed Tomography Facts, Controversy, and Future.* Nathan D. Wong, PhD; Robert C Detrano, MD, PhD; David Abrahamson, MD; Jonathan M Tobis, MD; Julius M Gardin, MD

Circulation. 2000;102:126. *American College of Cardiology/American Heart Association Expert Consensus Document on Electron-Beam Computed Tomography for the Diagnosis and Prognosis of Coronary - ACC/AHA Expert Consensus Document.* http://circ.ahajournals.org/cgi/content/full/102/1/126

Circulation. 2001;104(14):1682-87 (ISSN: 1524-4539). *Unstable coronary plaque and its relation to coronary calcium.* Schmermund A; Erbel R

Cleveland Clinic Journal of Medicine. June 2005;Vol 22(6):487-95 (ISSN 0891-1150). *Intravascular Ultrasonography; Using Endpoints in Coronary Atherosclerosis Trials.* Paul Schoenhagen, MD; Steven E Nissen, MD

Clinical Cardiology. 1999;22:554-558. *Electron Beam Computed Tomography: Screening for Coronary Artery Disease.* Matthew J Budoff, MD; and Bruce H Brundage, MD

Ethnicity and Disease. 2005;15(2):198-204 (ISSN: 1 049-510X). *Race-ethnic differences in the extent, prevalence, and progression of coronary calcium.* Kawakubo M, LaBree L, Xiang M, Doherty TM, Wong ND, Azen S, Detrano R

European Radiology. 2005;15(1):96-101 (ISSN: 0938-7994). *CT measurement of coronary calcium mass: impact on global cardiac risk assessment.* Becker CR; Majeed A; Crispin A; Knez A; Schoepf UJ; Boekstegers P; Steinbeck G; Reiser MF

Herz. 2001;26(4):278-86 (ISSN: 0340-9937). *Progression of coronary calcium.* Schmermund, A

Journal of Clinical Outcomes Management. 2001;Vol 8(11). *Prognostic Value of Coronary Artery Calcification.* Matthew J Budoff MD

Journal of the American College of Cardiology. 2001;37(6):1506-11 (ISSN: 0735-1097). *Electron Beam Tomography and National Cholesterol Education Program Guidelines in Asymptomatic Women.* Heecht HS; Superko HR

Journal of the American Medical Association. Jan 14, 2004;Vol 291(2). *Coronary Artery Calcium Score Combined With Framingham Score for Risk Prediction in Asymptomatic Individuals.* Philip Greenland, MD; Laurie LaBree,

MS; Stanley P. Azen, PhD; Terence M. Doherty, BA; Robert C. Detrano, MD, PhD

Los Angeles Times. Sept 2003. *Peace of Mind – But At a Price – Elective CT Scans.* Daniel Costello

Mayo Clinic Proceedings. 1996;71:369-377. *Electron Beam Computed Tomography and Coronary Artery Disease: Scanning for Coronary Artery Calcification.* John A Rumberger, MD, PHD; Patrick F Sheedy II, MD; Jerome F Breen, MD; Lorraine A Fitzpatrick, MD; and Robert S Schwartz, MD

The New York Times. November 26, 1995; Vol CXLV(50256). *Tests Detect Heart Problems in People Who Seem Healthy.* Gina Kolata

The Wall Street Journal. February 8, 1998. *Ads for Heart Scans Prompt Wider Use of Helpful Screening.* Marilyn Chase

USA Today. June 22, 1999. *Keys to Life; Manual Typewriter, Heartscan - One enriched Life, the Other Saved It.* Senator Paul Simon

Zeitschrift für Kardiologie. 2001; 90(1):21-7 (ISSN: 0300-5860). [Exclusion of coronary calcium with electron beam tomography: an effective filter before invasive diagnosis in symptomatic patients?] Haberl R, Becker A, Lang C, Becker C, Knez A, Leber A, Bruning R, Reiser M, Steinbeck G

Chapter 15

A couple of comprehensive sites about Aortic Aneurysm disease. A very long address for the second page, but worth the typing.
   http://www.medicinenet.com/abdominal_aortic_aneurysm/article.htm
   http://www.vascularweb.org/_CONTRIBUTION_PAGES/
   Patient_Information/NorthPoint/Abdominal_Aortic_Aneursym.html

Agency for Healthcare Research and Quality (AHRQ). Publication No. 05-0569-C Preventive Services Task Force - *Cost-Effectiveness Analyses of Population-Based Screening for Abdominal Aortic Aneurysm: Evidence Synthesis.* Richard T Meenan, PhD, MPHA; Craig Fleming, MDA; Evelyn P Whitlock, MD, MPHA; Tracy L Beil, MSA; Paula Smith, BSNA

American Family Physician. April 1, 2006; Vol 73(7). *Abdominal Aortic Aneurysm.* Gilbert R Upchurch, JR., MD; and Timothy A Schaub, MD; University of Michigan Health System, Ann Arbor, Michigan

Annals of Internal Medicine. Feb 2005; Vol 142(3):198-202. *Screening for Abdominal Aortic Aneurysm: Recommendation Statement.* United States Preventive Services Task Force

Internal Medicine News. Aug 15, 2005; Vol 38(16). *Extreme Emotions, Exertion Can Spur Aortic Ruptures – Expert Urges Echo Exams as a Preventive.* Bruce Jancin

The Society of Thoracic Surgeons. *Aortic Aneurysm* – review article
http://www.sts.org/sections/patientinformation/aneurysmsurgery/
aorticaneurysms/index.html

United States Preventive Services Task Force (USPSTF) guidelines *Screening for Abdominal Aortic Aneurysm* – Release Date: 2005 http://www.ahrq.gov/clinic/uspstf/uspsaneu.htm

Chapter 16

American Journal of Medicine. 2005;118:1067-77. *Low HDL-C: A Secondary Target of Dyslipidemia Therapy.* Robert S Rosenson, MD

Arteriosclerosis, Thrombosis, and Vascular Biology. 2005;25:1-7. *Low-Density Lipoprotein Subfractions and the Long-Term Risk of Ischemic Heart Disease in Men - 13-year Follow-Up Data From the Quebec Cardiovascular Study.* Annie C St-Pierre, Bernard Cantin, Gilles R Dagenais, Pascale Mauriège, Paul Marie Bernard, Jean-Pierre Desprès, Bonoît Lamarche

Atherosclerosis. 2004;174(1):93-8. *Rosuvastatin reduces MMP-7 secretion by human monocyte-derived macrophages: potential relevance to atherosclerotic plaque stability.* Furman C, Copin C, Kandoussi M, Davidson R., Moreau M, McTaggiar F, Chapman MJ, Fruchart JC, Rouis M.

Baylor College of Medicine Reports on Cardiometabolic Disorders. Vol 1(1). *Assessing the Patient for Cardiometabolic Risk.* Peter H Jones, MD; Christie M Ballantyne, MD

Berkeley Heart Lab—a major innovator in the fine-tuning of blood lipid analysis. http://www.berkeleyheartlab.com/

British Medical Journal. May 2006;6(332):1064-7. *Active and Passive Smoking and Development of Glucose Intolerance Among Young Adults in a Progressive Cohort.* Houston TK, et al.

Circulation. 2001; 04:2295-99. *Comparison of Various Electrophoretic Characteristics of LDL Particles and Their Relationship to the Risk of Ischemic Heart Disease.* AC St-Pierre, BSc; I.L. Ruel, BSc; B Cantin, MD, PhD; GR Dagenais, MD; PM Bernard, MSc; JP Despres, PhD; B Lamarche, PhD

Current Drug Targets. Mar 2005;6(2):215-23. *Cannabinoids and the regulation of ingestive behaviour.* Vickers SP, Kennett GA.

Diabetes Care. Jan 2004;Vol 27(Supp 1). *Standards of Medical Care in Diabetes.* American Diabetes Association

Diabetes Consult Collection. April 2006:5-6. *Clinical Use of Exenatide: The First of a New Class of Incretin Mimetics.* Daniel A Nadeau, MD

Diabetes Consult Collection. April 2006:7-9. *Clinical Effects of Incretin Mimetic and Amylin Analog Hormones.* Leonel Villa-Caballero, MD; Steven V

Edelman, MD

Diabetes Forecast. April 2006. *Cholesterol Drug (Fenofibrate) Has Multiple Benefits.* Terri D'Arrigo

Diabetologia. 2005;48(Suppl):A410-11,Abs 1137. *Anti-atherosclerotic and renoprotective effects of rosuvastatin in a model of diabetes- accelerated atherosclerosis.* Jandeleit Dahm KAM, Giunti S, Boolell v, Calkin A, Lassila M, Allen TJ, Cooper ME.

DOCNews. July 2006. *New American Diabetic Association Initiative Moves Beyond 'Metabolic Syndrome.'* Elizabeth Thompson Beckley

Emergency Medicine. Jan 2006;Vol 38(1):22-30. *The Evidence in Favor of Lipid Management.* Marc S Itskowitz, MD, FACP

Internal Medicine News. Vol 39(14). *Rimonabant Tied to Blood Pressure Drop in Obesity.* Eric Goldman

Internal Medicine World Report. May 2006;Vol 21(5). *State-of-the-Art Diabetes Management.* Laura Brasseur

International Journal of Clinical Practice. 2005;59(Suppl.148):10-11. *Rosuvastatin enhances arteriogenesis in a murine disease model of apoE-/- deficiency.* Hoefer I, Hedwig F, Meder B, Ulusans S, Bergmann C, Fischer S, van Royen N, Buschmann I.

Johns Hopkins Medicine - Cardiology News and Issues in the New Millennium. Vol 4(7). *Large LDL and HDL Particles Are Associated with Longevity.* Ty Gluckman, MD; Nove Kalia, MBBS

Johns Hopkins Medicine – Cardiology News and Issues in the New Millennium. Vol 4(1). *HDL and ApoA-1 Are Key Therapeutic Targets In Novel Treatments for Atherosclerosis.* Navin Kapur, MD; Khurram Nasir, MD

Johns Hopkins Medicine – Cardiology News and Issues in the New Millennium. Vol 4(1). *The New Challenge of Managing HDL and Triglycerides.* Nove Kalia, MBBS

Journal De Pharmacie De Belgique. 2005;60(3):89-91. *Rimonabant (Acomplia), specific inhibitor of the endocannabinoid system.* [Article in French] Ducobu J, Sternon J, CHU Tivoli, La Louviere, ULB.

Lipidletter. Dec 2005;Vol 5(2). *Metabolic Syndrome in the Clinic: focus on Visceral Obesity and Triglycerides.* L Marie Belalcazar, MD

Lipidletter. March 2005;Vol 4(3). *What Do We Know About Pleiotropic Effects (of statins).* Scott Kinlay, MBBS, PhD

Chapter 17

A few cigarettes a day 'deadly' – Story from BBC NEWS: http://news.bbc.co.uk/go/pr/fr/-/1/hi/health/4265600.stm Published: 2005/09/22 00:00:40 GMT

American Journal of Respiratory and Critical Care Medicine. 2005;Vol 171:1378-83. *Early Lung Cancer Detection Using Spiral Computed Tomography and Positron Emission Tomography.* Gorka Bastarrika, Maria Jose Garcia-Velloso, Maria Dolores Lozano, Usua Montes, Wenceslao Torre, Natalia Spiteri, Arantza Campo, Luis Seijo, Ana Belen Alcaide, Jesus Pueyo, David Cano, Isabel Vivas, Octavio Cosin, Pablo Dominguez, Patricia Serra, Jose A Richter, Luis Montuenga, and Javier J Zulueta

Cornell medical college to receive $3.6 Million for CT screening research – Cornell News, April 26, 2004.

Journal of the American Medical Association. 2006;Vol 296. *Effect of Maintenance Therapy With Varenicline on Smoking Cessation A Randomized Controlled Trial.* Serena Tonstad, MD, PhD; Philip Tønnesen, MD, PhD; Peter Hajek, PhD; Kathryn E Williams, PhD; Clare B Billing, MS; Karen R Reeves, MD; for the Varenicline Phase 3 Study Group

Journal of the American Medical Association. 2006;Vol 296. *Varenicline, an a4β2 Nicotinic Acetylcholine Receptor Partial Agonist, vs Sustained-Release Bupropion and Placebo for Smoking Cessation – A Randomized Controlled Trial.* David Gonzales, PhD; Stephen I Rennard, MD; Mitchell Nides, PhD; Cheryl Onck~n, MD; Salomon Azoulay, MD; Clare B Billing, MS; Eric J Watsky, MD; Jason Gong, MD; Kathryn E Williams, PhD; Karen R Reeves, MD

Journal of the American Medical Association. 2006;Vol 296. *Efficacy of Varenicline, an a4β2 Nicotinic Acetylcholine receptor Partial Agonist, vs Placebo or Sustained-Release Bupropion for smoking Cessation – A Randomized controlled trial.* Douglas E Jorenby, PhD; J. Taylor Hays, MD; Nancy A Rigotti, MD; Salomon Azoulay, MD; Eric J Watsky, MD; Kathryn E Williams, PhD; Clare B Billing, MS; Jason Gong, MD; Karen R Reeves, MD

Lung cancer prevention and screening. Jess Mandel, MD

Research shows smoking one cigarette affects heart – East Carolina University, Office of News and Information

Smoking Dangers. Garret Condon

The latest information to help people quit smoking, and to help healthcare professionals treat tobacco use and dependence. http://www.surgeongeneral.gov/tobacco/

United States Preventive Services Task Force (USPSTF) *Summary of Recommendations for Lung Cancer Screening.*

Chapter 18

American Journal of Medicine. 2005;118:1078-88. *Screening for Colorectal, Breast and Cervical Cancer in the Elderly: A Review of the Evidence.* Louise C Walter, MD; Carmen L Lewis, MD, MPH; Mary B Barton, MD, MPP

ACS Screening guidelines – *Colon Cancer*

New England Journal of Medicine. Dec 4, 2003;349:23. *Computed Tomographic Virtual Colonoscopy to Screen for Colorectal Neoplasia in Asymptomatic Adults.* Perry J Pickhardt, MD; J Richard Choi, ScD, MD; Inku Hwang, MD; James A Butler, MD; Michaell. Puckett, MD; Hans A Hildebrandt, MD; Roy K Wong, MD; Pamela A Nugent, MD; Pauline A Mysliwiec, MD, MPH; and William R Schindler, DO

The Jay Monahan Center for Gastrointestinal health. http://www.monahancenter.org/

United States Preventive Services Task Force (USPSTF) *Summary of Recommendations for Colon Cancer Screening.*

Chapter 19

A resource to evaluate issues surrounding Prostate Cancer and its screening. http://www.cdc.gov/cancer/prostate/publications/decisionguide/

ACS Screening Guidelines: *Prostate Cancer.*

Archives of Internal Medicine. 2006;166:38-43. *The Effectiveness of Screening for Prostate Cancer.* John Concato, MD, MPH; Carolyn K Wells, MPH; Ralph I Horwitz, MD; David Penson, MD; Graeme Fincke, MD; Dan R Berlowitz, MD, MPH; Gregory Froehlich, MD; Dawna Blake, MD; Martyn A Vickers, MD; Gerald A Gehr, MD; Nabil H Raheb, MD; Gail Sullivan, MD, MPH; Peter Peduzzi, PhD

Cleveland Clinic Journal of Medicine. June 2005;Vol 22(6):521-27. (ISSN 0891-1150) *Prostate-Specific Antigen: How to advise Patients as the Screening Debate Continues.* Peter C. Albertsen, MD, MS

Internal Medicine News. Vol 39(12). *Guidelines Grapple With Localized Prostate Cancer.* Fran Lowry

Johns Hopkins Medical Institutions. May 16, 2005. *New Test for Early Detection of Prostate Cancer Shows Promise* and *Novel prostate cancer marker may lead to earlier diagnosis and fewer repeat biopsies.* Study results appear in the May 15, 2005 issue of *Cancer Research.* The lead author is Robert H Getzenberg, PhD

New England Journal of Medicine. Sep 22, 2005;Vol 353(12):1224-35. *Autoantibody Signatures in Prostate Cancer.* First author: Xiaoju Wang, PhD, University of Michigan Medical School.

Proceedings from the 2006 annual meeting of the American Urological Association. May 2006. Abstract #851. *EPCA plus PSA Highly Accurate in Detecting Prostate Cancer.*

Prostate Biopsy calculator http://www.compass.fhcrc.org/edrnnci/bin/calculator/main.asp

The Journal of Family Practice. July 2005;Vol 54(7):586-96. *Screening For Prostate cancer, Who and how often.*

Time Magazine. April 1, 1996. *The Man's Cancer: Prostate cancer is reaching epidemic levels in the U.S.* General Norman Schwarzkopf

United States Preventive Services Task Force (USPSTF) *Summary of Recommendations for Prostate Cancer Screening.*

Chapter 20

ACS Screening Guidelines: *Breast Cancer.*

An interactive breast cancer risk assessment tool can be found at this page of the National Cancer Institute Website http://www.cancer.gov/bcrisktool/

Another helpful website by Steven B Halls, MD. http://www.halls.md/breast/risk.htm

Internal Medicine News. May 15, 2006;Vol 39(10). *Raloxifene Works For Prevention of Invasive Breast Cancer – Risk reduction comparable to tamoxifen.* Robert Finn

Internal Medicine News. Vol 39(1). *Statins May Curb ER-Negative Breast Cancer Risk.* Bruce Jancin

New England Journal of Medicine. 2004;351:427-37, 497-500. *Efficacy of MRI and Mammography for Breast-Cancer Screening in Women with a Familial or Genetic Predisposition.* Mieke Kriege, M.Sc.; Cecile TM Brekelmans, MD, PhD; Carla Boetes, MD, PhD; Peter E Besnard, MD, PhD; Harmine M Zonderland, MD, PhD; Inge Marie Obdeijn, MD; Radu A Manoliu, MD, PhD; Theo Kok, MD, PhD; Hans Peterse, MD; Madeleine MA Tilanus-Linthorst, MD; Sara H Muller, MD, PhD; Sybren Meijer, MD, PhD; Jan C Oosterwijk, MD, PhD; Louk VAM Beex, MD, PhD; Rob AEM Tollenaar, MD, PhD; Harry J de Koning, MD, PhD; Emiel JT Rutgers, MD, PhD; Jan GM Klijn, MD, PhD; for the Magnetic Resonance Imaging Screening Study Group

Postgraduate Medicine. Aug 2005;Vol 118(2). *Breast Cancer Screening –Benefits, Risks and Current Controversies*. Mary B Barton, MD, MPP

Postgraduate Medicine. Aug 2005;Vol 118(2). *What's the deal With Menopause Management – Why the Women's Health Initiative Raises More Questions Than It Answers* Marcie K Richardson MD

Stanford School of Medicine. April 11, 2006 - News Release. *No Link Between*

Estrogen-Only Therapy, Breast Cancer in Postmenopausal Women. http:/
/mednews.stanford.edu/releases/2006/april/estrogen.html

The Bend Bulletin. May 2003. *Hormone Replacement Therapy May Be Good
For Some Women* John L Corso, MD

United States Preventive Services Task Force (USPSTF) *Summary of Recommendations for BRCA Testing.*

United States Preventive Services Task Force (USPSTF) *Summary of Recommendations for Breast Cancer Screening.*

Chapter 21

American Family Physician. 2006;73:2187-94. *Esophageal Cancer: A Review
and Update.* John C Layke, DO; Peter P Lopez, MD

American Family Physician. 2006;73:2195-200. *Management of Hip Fracture:
The Family Physician's Role.* Shoba S Rao, MD; Manjula Cherukuri, MD

American Family Physician. February 1, 2004. *Treatment of Obstructive Sleep
Apnea in Primary Care.* Lyle D Victor, MD, MBA

American Family Physician. July 15, 2005;Vol 72(2). *Cutaneous Melanoma: Update on Prevention, Screening, Diagnosis and Treatment.* Brika L Rager,
MD, MPH; Edward P Bridgeford, MD; David W Ollila, MD

American Journal of Public Health. May 1988;78(5):544-47. *Sleep apnea and
mortality in an aged cohort.* DL Bliwise, NG Bliwise, M Partinen, AM Pursley,
and WC Dement

American Sleep Apnea Association. http://www.sleepapnea.org/

Bladder Cancer information The Mayo Clinic website. http://www.mayoclinic.com/
health/bladder-cancer/DS00177

Consultant. Nov 2005;Vol 45(13). *Waking Up to Insomnia: A significant Problem.* Karl Doghramji, MD

e-Medicine - Web MD. *Obstructive Sleep Apnea Syndrome.* Andrew J Lipton,
MD, MPH and TM, Staff Pediatric Pulmonologist, Assistant Professor of
Pediatrics, Department of Pediatrics, Walter Reed Army Medical Center. http:/
/www.emedicine.com/ped/byname/obstructive-sleep-apnea-syndrome.htm

e-Medicine - Web MD. *Malignant Melanoma.* Susan M Swetter, MD, Director,
Pigmented Lesion and Cutaneous Melanoma Clinic, Associate Professor,
Department of Dermatology, Stanford University Medical Center/VA Palo
Alto Health Care System http://www.emedicine.com/derm/byname/malignant-
melanoma.htm

e-Medicine - Web MD. *Osteoporosis.* Julie Lin, MD; Joseph M Lane, MD; http:/

/www.emedicine.com/orthoped/topic240.htm

Family Practice News. June 15, 2000. *Sleep Apnea Symptoms Differ in Women vs. Men.* by Mitchel L Zoler

HPV vaccination news from the National Cancer Institute. http://www.cancer.gov/clinicaltrials/results/cervical-cancer-vaccine1102

Internal Medicine News Vol 39(12). *Prevalence of HPV Peaks in 14- to 19-Year-Old Females.* Damian McNamara

Internal Medicine News. Vol 39(12). *HPV Vaccine Wins Strong Support.* Elizabeth Machcatie

Johns Hopkins Advanced Studies in Medicine. May 2006;Vol 6(5). *Early Ovarian Cancer; Prevention, Diagnosis, Treatment.* Lee-may Chen, MD

Journal of Clinical Endocrinology and Metabolism. Nov 2002;87:4914-23. *Effect of discontinuation of estrogen, calcitriol, and the combination of both on bone density and bone markers.* Gallagher JC, et al.

Journal of the American Academy of Dermatology. 1998;Vol 39:262-67. *Use of Dermatologic Photography to Aid Surveillance of Individuals At High Risk for Melanoma.* Arthur R Rhodes, MD, MPH

Journal of the American Medical Association. 2002; 288:321 *Changes in Bone Density After Stopping HRT*

Journal of the American Medical Association. 2005;294:2052-56. *Measurement level of telomerase activity in urine may help detect bladder cancer in men.*

Malignant Melanoma information from the American Academy of Dermatology http://www.aad.org/public/Publications/pamphlets/MalignantMelanoma.htm

National Osteoporosis Foundation website. http://www.nof.org/

New England Journal of Medicine. Nov 10, 2005;Vol 353(19):2034-41. *Obstructive Sleep Apnea as a Risk Factor for Stroke and Death.* H Klar Yaggi, MD, MPH; John Concato, MD, MPH; Walter N Kernan, MD; Judith H Lichtman, PhD, MPH; Lawrence M Brass, MD; and Vahid Mohsenin, MD

NewScientist.com News Service. April 18, 2005. *Will cancer vaccine get to all women?* Debora MacKenzie http://www.newscientist.com/channel/sex/mg18624954.500

NIH Osteoporosis and Related Bone Diseases ~ National Resource Center website. http://www.niams.nih.gov/bone/

Postgraduate Medicine. Aug 2005;Vol 118(2). *Pap Tests and HPV Infection – Advances in Screening and Interpretation.* Elizabeth J Buechler

Proceedings Of The National Academy Of Sciences Of The United States Of

America. May 24, 2005;102:7677-82. ***Serum Protein Markers for Early Detection of Ovarian Cancer.*** Mor G, et al.

United States Preventive Services Task Force (USPSTF) ***Summary of Recommendations for Bladder Cancer Screening.***

United States Preventive Services Task Force (USPSTF) ***Summary of Recommendations for Cervical Cancer Screening.***

INDEX

Acknowledgements

Just as I was wrapping up a health talk, called *Dumb Reasons to Die*, at our local Senior Center, a thoughtful, older gentleman came up from the audience to tell me I should write a book—a book on the same health subjects and, more importantly, in the same *everyday language* as my lecture. He thanked me, not so much for what I was teaching, but for how I was able to teach it. So I began writing.

That was 1997. But writing a book I'd be willing to put my name to turned out to be a bit harder than I expected. It's taken nine years, many false starts and, above all, a supportive and talented team of helpers to pull it off.

Debi, my dear wife and partner in all things, without your enthusiastic and active pursuit of our mission—to really and truly save lives by empowering individual patients—this project would be nowhere. You created the space I needed to put on paper the lessons of my medical practice, and then you took on the thousands of details that turn a manuscript into a book, web site, and lecture series. How happy and fortunate I am to share my life with you.

Amie and Anthony, next to Mom you are at the top of my thank-you list for putting up with my distraction and obsession over the past year. Because you are both so bright, positive, and helpful, I've had the environment at home to finish this project. How did we get so lucky in our children? Anyway, thank you both for not shooting me.

Vicki Grant, you are my writing soul mate. Never has collaboration felt more effortless. Are you this creative, responsive and dead-on in all your writing? I'd only consider starting another book knowing *you'd be there* to improve everything I said.

Cynthia Stark, you're my lifeline—an expert guide in a dangerous land. (Did I use the Em Dash correctly just then? Oh, and sorry about these parentheses.) Your eagle-eye for consistency, clarity, and all manner of detail is humbling. And that's not counting your tireless efforts to keep me out of dangerous traps, both legal *and* grammatical.

Mark Blackwell, what can I say? Whenever I think of how I almost *didn't* ask you to illustrate this book, assuming you were just too busy, I break out in a cold sweat. I can never thank you enough for the talent, wit and the heroic effort you brought to bear on this project, under such enormous time pressure. What joy receiving your emails!

Shannon Cooper, you are my right *and* left arm in all things medical. Without the dedication, reliability, initiative and sheer joy you bring to our medical practice and every patient in it, I would never have felt the peace of mind I needed to complete this book. If you ever retire, I may have to follow suit.

Jim Cajacob and Cal Mukumoto, thank you for your creative wisdom, ongoing collaboration, and valued friendship. To author and friend, Leslie Godwin, and her house guest, Petey, my deepest thanks for all your constructive editing, content suggestions, and ongoing enthusiasm for this project. Thanks to Steve Worshtil for cutting out so much junk and helping me get back on track, to Kirsten Goldstein for your infectious enthusiasm and support, and to Dru Johnson, for being not only my coach, but the cheerleader in my corner when I needed one. Thanks to my dear friend, Katie Merritt, for landing what amounts to a verbal slap up side my head two years ago—that's what real friends are for.

I had the great fortune to be born into one of the happiest and more functional families of the Baby-Boomer generation. Credit for that, of course, goes to my late, beloved mother, Jane, and my dear father, Louis, and to all my brothers and sisters, nieces and nephews and in-laws. I treasure you all.

That leaves everyone else, too many to mention, who have encouraged and tolerated me throughout this project. Among them a very special thanks goes out to all my own patients at the Personal Access Program of High Lakes Health Care, and to all my patients over the last twenty years, for sharing with me your lives, your friendship, your stories, and your trust.

Oh, and thanks to the gentleman who made the effort to encourage me nine years ago at the senior center. That was a nice thing to do.

∼∼∼